UNDERSTANDING YOGA

By the same author

YOGA AND THE BHAGAVAD-GITA

UNDERSTANDING
YOGA

A Thematic Companion to Yoga and Indian Philosophy

Tom McArthur

Illustrated by Steinar Lund

THE AQUARIAN PRESS
Wellingborough, Northamptonshire

First published 1986

To the organizers and members
of the Scottish Yoga Association,
past, present and prospective

British Library Cataloguing in Publication Data

McArthur, Tom
   Understanding yoga: A thematic
   companion to yoga and Indian
   philosophy
   1. Yoga
   I. Title
   181'.45   B132.Y6

   ISBN 0-85030-479-2

*The Aquarian Press is part of the
Thorsons Publishing Group*

Printed and bound in Great Britain

Contents

Preface

This is a book that looks at yoga through language. It deals in themes and key expressions like *asana*, *ashram*, *chakra*, *guru*, *mantra*, *maya*, and *prana*—expressions that one cannot escape from in any inquiry into the subject. In addition, it looks at yoga in terms of such other areas of interest, belief and dogma as 'science', 'religion', 'the occult', 'magic', 'health and fitness', and 'mysticism'. In the process, it covers a large number of terms and ideas originating in Sanskrit, as well as trying to clarify an equally wide range of expressions currently circulating in English and particularly in books about yoga.

Organized in thematic form, it also has a detailed index to help users locate definitions and descriptions of words and ideas that belong in, and across, the themes chosen. In effect, you can read the book from start to finish, or start with the theme that interests you most, or even go to the index first and choose a term. In this way, it can serve as a companion, to be read, re-read, and dipped into as the need arises.

The present form and content of *Understanding Yoga* have emerged out of an alphabetic glossary that I created for the use of students attending courses in Indian philosophy, religion, and yoga that I ran in the 1970s for the Department of Extra-Mural Studies at the University of Edinburgh, in broad collaboration with the Scottish Yoga Association. Many people took part in these courses and in related seminars that drew participants from all over Scotland, helping me to frame the issues more clearly in my own mind. Among those people I would like to acknowledge in particular Patricia Bramah, George Chalmers, Violet Henderson, Margaret Hendry, Helen Hogg, Feri McArthur, Patti McTavish, William Mowat-Thomson, Ian Scorgie, and Jane Thomson, for all their help, advice, support and encouragement. Margaret Hendry and Feri McArthur are specially to be thanked, for their help in creating the final shape of this book.

Introduction

Suppose you read an academic book about yoga, and in it you come across the word *saṁsara*—mysterious dot above the 'm' and all. Then a week or two later you happen to attend a discourse given by an Indian swami who talks about the wheel of birth and death, and several times includes a word that sounds like *sangsar*.

There is no reason to suppose that they are the same word, and nobody is likely to enlighten you about them. Additionally, in the same general context you could come across the term *saṁskara*, and wonder where it fits in. It is not at all the same word, but that isn't easy to check either. And if you find it in an academic book with the dot *below* the 'm' (as can happen), what are you to make of *that*? Simpler, perhaps, just to ignore it.

I could have chosen other examples; there are plenty. I chose these, however, because all three gave me problems at one time, and took me quite a while to sort out. An interested Westerner faces such difficulties all the time with the Sanskrit terms of yoga—as regards both pronunciation and the armoury of little marks that scholars use when putting Sanskrit into the roman alphabet. As more and more Sanskrit expressions come into English, and as people consult a wider range of sources that have incorporated the Indian terms into English in different ways at different times, the problems increase rather than decrease.

This could be called the front line of difficulty when people are reading about, and teaching, yoga. In spite of the great number of books currently available on the subject, there is little direct help on matters like these.

The first aim of this book, therefore, is to help at this basic level of language mystification. To do this, I have provided a section which deals with Sanskrit in English, then scattered through the whole book background information on a large number of words regularly used in yoga circles. There is also an index.

The second aim, however, goes beyond the basic uses and meanings of words—how to pronounce them (more or less), how to spell them, and how to recognize their variations. I have also tried to provide something of the flavour of Sanskrit, as well as an insight into the worldview that has pervaded both Sanskrit and yoga during some three thousand years. To do this, I have grouped words, ideas, stories, and comment thematically, under certain 'key' expressions, in order to show how these have evolved, and how different people and schools of thought have used and interpreted them. Many books on yoga provide glossaries that define such terms concisely, but they do not explore their cultural range or discuss the controversies that frequently surround them. I am thinking here of words like *asana*, *chakra*, and *prana*, which can mean different things to different people, and badly need some critical analysis.

Thirdly, I am also interested in the kinds of people who produce books on yoga, both in India and in the West. Knowing something about them and about their backgrounds is useful in understanding the key terms of the subject, because different writers with different aims use the same terms in different ways. Although the goal of yoga is often described as integration and unification, the language of yoga is not a unity. All books everywhere are biassed, whether obviously or subtly—this one included. All authors take certain things for granted, and neglect to enlarge upon them. This is as true of yoga books as any others, and quite often what writers have taken for granted and not discussed is precisely what their readers need to know in order to make informed judgements and decisions. This book is an attempt to bring the 'taken for granted' of yoga out into the open for a closer examination.

Books on yoga are varied, but fall into six broad categories, which can mean at least six areas of possible bias and at least six backgrounds to consider. These categories are:

1. The original Sanskrit texts, untranslated, of such works as the *Bhagavad-Gita*, the *Yoga-sutras*, and the *Hatha-yoga Pradipika*. These cannot simply be swallowed whole, and need to be seen against the background of their times and of their language of expression, Sanskrit.

2. Commentaries on these texts by Hindus, either in Sanskrit, or in a modern Indian language, or in English. Where one deals with these, one has to ask who wrote the commentary, when and where, and why.

3. Translations (wholly or in part, literally or in adapted form) of the

original texts (and commentaries) into Western languages like English, German and French. These have been done mainly by Westerners with their separate understandings of Sanskrit, and with their own reasons for making the translations, and for adding any commentaries of their own.

4. Books—mainly manuals of one kind or another—both by Hindus and Westerners with an interest in the occult. This interest might range from theosophy and 'the perennial philosophy' on the one side through assumptions about certain age-old 'secret doctrines' to assertions about Lost Civilizations and Hidden Masters who guide the human race. In such books, yoga is generally conceived as belonging by right in the occult domain.

5. Books—mainly works of history, anthropology, literature, language, and philosophy—by Western or Westernized Indian academics that seek to create more or less objective pictures of Indian philosophy, religion and yoga. These works share a desire for 'scholarly rigour' and are often animated by the spirit of scientific caution, if not a defensive scepticism.

6. Books—mainly manuals of health and self-improvement—both by Westerners and by Indians who have Western audiences in mind. These focus in the main on the physical, psychological, and therapeutic aspects of yoga and may incorporate more or less adeptly elements of Western anatomy, physiology, and medical science. They are 'how-to' books, whose authors are variously qualified in the areas which they discuss.

There can be plenty of overlap too, of course. Between the same covers, for example, we might find a translation from an original source such as Patanjali, some commentary on it, an assertion that yoga is 'an ancient life science' (without making it clear what the phrase might mean), the use of Western anatomical and physiological descriptions of a physical pose beside Eastern mystical interpretations (without much attempt to harmonize the two), and the observation that Jesus Christ was a Yogi (without necessarily then making the case for his being one). The range of possibilities between the covers of yoga books is considerable.

In books like these, it is not always easy for a reader to be sure of what is going on: whether the writer is speaking for all yogis and kinds of yoga, whether assertions that something has been 'proved scientifically' are justified or not, or whether a particular view of the world belongs to yoga at large, to a particular group, or to the private speculations and convictions of the writer alone. The frame of reference may well be clear to the writer, who sees his or her subject whole and has lived with it for years, but may be unclear to the reader—and unsettling as well.

This book is intended therefore for people who would like to know a bit more about the packages of ideas and actions that they are being asked to buy: what the ideologies are, where the evangelism lies, and which viewpoints are whose, especially as regards the essential terminology of the subject. It offers no absolute conclusions, but does I hope display the options and the angles of vision. If some of those options and angles are bewildering, even after a deal of explanation, then the reader will know that I at least cannot make them any simpler, after having tried to do so for some twenty years or more.

My fourth and final aim is the simplest of them all. This is a book about yoga, but approached from the angle of language rather than of physical fitness, philosophy, or cosmic consciousness. These all crowd in, of course, but they are not the *darshana* of the book. The language viewpoint may, however, prove helpful, and certainly enables me to tell some of my favourite stories while analysing the key words of yoga.

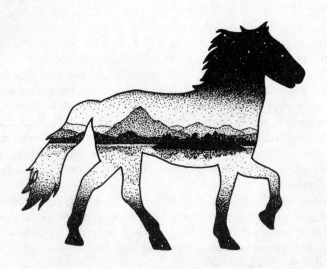

1. Sanskrit in English

Dhritarashtra uvacha:
Dharma-kshetre kuru-kshetre samaveta yuyutsavah
mamakah Pandavash ch'aiva: kim akurvata, Samjaya?

That is Sanskrit, the first three lines in fact of the *Bhagavad-Gita*, where Dhritarashtra asks: 'Sanjaya, what did they do, all my men and the sons of Pandu, when they were marshalled for the fight, on the field of duty, on the field of the Kurus?'

Here, the word *dharma* is translated as 'duty', which is a fair translation but hardly catches the enormous significance of *dharma* to the Hindu mind. If the word is translated every time it appears, the reader never meets it directly and cannot come to terms with it as a key word of yoga in the *Gita*. In my own version of the *Gita* I have tried to bring such terms into the text alongside suitable translation equivalents—to help the reader see what the compiler was seeing. In the process I have of course seeded English with Sanskrit, as others have done and are doing. This I think is necessary and inevitable, just as the musical vocabulary of English is seeded with Italian. To let *dharma* lie unseen behind such translations as 'duty' and 'order' is to some extent a misrepresentation of what is going on. One needs to make such words as visible as possible.

Sanskrit is a difficult language to learn, and few people now learn it, either in India or in the West. This does not mean, however, that one cannot acquire a technical vocabulary of Sanskrit-in-English much as a musician learns the Italian terms of music. Sanskrit is remoter than Italian, of course, particularly because it is normally written in the devanagari script ('the divine, civilized script'). This is a distant cousin of the roman alphabet, but hangs rather than sits on the line. In addition, each of its units is a syllable rather than a letter, which takes quite a lot of getting used to. Additionally, Sanskrit has a grammar like Latin and

Greek, and not too many people nowadays enjoy a tussle with classical languages. They may well feel that handling their own language and maybe *one* other modern language is enough to take on in a busy life, without going in for 'dead' languages as well.

Thirdly, and importantly, Sanskrit is difficult because of the worldview that lies behind the words and the grammar. Even people who find yoga immensely attractive and who have travelled widely in India from time to time come up against something that jars them culturally: a statement, a text, or a story that strains sympathy to its limit, or that the mind refuses to handle. This is true of present-day India, and is truer still of such works of the ancient Indian mind as the Vedas and the Upanishads. This is why translations made available to modern Western browsers are usually edited selections, not the whole of a text. Scholars have made choices in the effort to present something that can be enjoyed and understood (although never without an effort). The kind of thing they often leave out is the following, from the *Brihad-aranyaka Upanishad*:

Om! Verily, the dawn is the head of the sacrificial horse; the sun, his eye; the wind, his breath; universal fire his open mouth. The year is the body of the sacrificial horse; the sky, his back; the atmosphere, his belly; the earth, the underpart of his belly; the quarters, his flanks; the intermediate quarters, his ribs; the seasons his limbs; the months and half-months, his joints; days and nights, his feet; the stars, his bones; the clouds, his flesh. Sand is the food in his stomach; rivers are his entrails. His liver and lungs are the mountains; plants and trees, his hair. The orient is his fore part; the occident, his hind part. When he yawns, then it lightens. When he shakes himself, then it thunders. When he urinates, then it rains. Voice, indeed, is his voice.[1]

Some people would simply shrug at this and pass on; others might get a little poetic satisfaction from the excerpt. But nobody meditating on it is likely to grasp its essence in a flash of intuition. It is just too different for that. Yet Hindus see such material as a fundamental scriptural statement—even if they too have never read it or, having read it, have also failed to understand it. It is some consolation, however, that most scholars, East and West, consider this particular Upanishad both one of the earliest and one of the hardest to understand. It remains, nonetheless, part and parcel of the background of yoga.

It is of course couched in the language of myth, and this is one of the first things I want to talk about. Myth is the oldest means of explaining and describing serious issues, far older than reasoned discourse and scientific argument. Basic to myth is the idea of analogy, that what one finds hard to describe can be understood in terms of something more familiar. In this case the ancient sage chose an everyday creature, the horse, just as a modern swami might make his point by comparing life to a car. In addition, the horse analogy is tied to the idea of sacrifice, because animal sacrifices were common in those days—and human sacrifices not so far away either. The brahmin priests categorically believed at that time, something over 2,600 years ago, that their sacrifices were essential to the world: no sacrifices, no world. Furthermore, because the sacrifice of a horse was an expensive and rare spectacle, this sage used it as a powerful model for the whole universe.

'Imagine,' he was saying to his students as they sat at his feet, 'imagine that just as we now and again sacrifice a fine horse, so in the beginning the universe was formed from the body of a vast Cosmic Horse—but this horse was both a sacrifice and is still somehow alive.' After that, it was not so hard to match the universe part by part with the constituents and products of an animal everybody knew. Knowing this, we can even understand why rain should be equated with urine, and the Upanishad becomes a little less remote.

A student of yoga, however, has no more need to learn Sanskrit in order to grasp this kind of thing than a practising Christian has to learn Hebrew for the Old Testament and Greek for the New Testament of the Bible. At the same time, however, many words have come into English and other modern languages from those biblical sources, and the more one knows about 'shibboleth', 'cherub', 'exodus', and 'epistle' the better one's appreciation of what is in the Bible. In addition, the more we know about the Bible's equivalents of the Cosmic Horse, and about the societies in which such ideas grew up, the easier it is to adapt and apply such venerable images and ideas to modern times. They cease to be ancient, irrelevant nonsense that the up-to-date can shun, and they also cease to be deep mysteries that only the Initiated can explain to the Ignorant.

Sanskrit has actually been rubbing shoulders with languages like English for longer than one might suppose. Words like 'sugar' and 'candy' have Sanskrit connections, as have 'ginger', 'lacquer', and 'chintz'. When the British controlled India, they picked up Sanskrit terms and played with them, sometimes disdainfully and humorously, occasionally with grudging respect. *Pandita* ('learned') became 'pundit', adapted from the Hindu title for a wise man. For the British, however, a pundit had a specious wisdom, whence our current usages like 'political pundits' and 'TV pundits'. *Guru* is also something of a humorous term; like pundits, gurus should not, in the general view, be taken too seriously, and so when we read about 'gurus of the stock market' and 'management gurus' we know that the writer does not entirely trust **them.**

When the British saw the great wagon at Puri in Orissa they were impressed by its size and the fanaticism of its handlers. They were less impressed by the significance of *Jagannatha* ('Lord of the World'), the god to whom the wagon was dedicated. Wagon and god became 'juggernaut', and just as some Hindu fanatics threw themselves to be crushed under the wheels of the great wagon, so people are sometimes run over and killed in narrow English streets by juggernauts that roar past thatched cottages and 'ought to be banned'. The comparison is fair, but it is worth recalling that Jagannatha was another name for the god-man Krishna, who played the flute and chased the cow-girls—and drove Arjuna's chariot in the *Bhagavad-Gita*.

Sanskrit has existed for something like three times as long as English as we know it. It dates back, like yoga, at least three thousand years and has been revered as a high language since the days of the Vedic hymns, much as Europeans more recently revered Church Latin. The brahmins have always been proprietorial about Sanskrit, which means 'perfectly made' or 'completely done'; for them, it was the true mode of communion and communication between the gods in heaven and themselves, the gods on earth who mediated for the rest of humankind. Spoken Sanskrit was vastly more important than the written form, when it was finally—and grudgingly—adopted, and great weight was placed in brahminical ritual on getting the sounds right: get the sound wrong and you get the spell wrong; get the spell wrong, and the world could go wrong. It is out of this entirely magical and incantatory approach to their sacred language that the special concept of *mantra* emerged.

Hindus are conservative about Sanskrit and still stand in awe of it, much as many people in the West today are still in awe of classical Greek and Latin, although they might not freely admit to it. It is not surprising, therefore, that students of yoga worry about getting the pronunciation right if they use a Sanskrit term like *siddhasana*, and getting the spelling right if they are putting it down on paper. Bad enough getting the ancient spells wrong; worse, if you are also going to show yourself up as a 'yogic illiterate'. Better, many have concluded, simply to avoid the problem and use Western expressions instead, like the Perfect Pose.

The brahmins apparently loved Sanskrit to death. By turning it into the perfect tool for gods, they killed it as a dynamic social medium for human beings; it became a purely technical, literary, and ceremonial language. At one time it served as a common language of religion, philosophy and scholarship across India, but nowadays it is something of a fossil, its wider role usurped by English. Such blends of English and Sanskrit as 'yogic', 'advaitic', and even 'post-Upanishadic' (which are in fact blends of Sanskrit, Latin, and Greek elements *in* English) are on the increase as scholars, Eastern and Western, continue to delve into the Hindu past and make their findings available to the widest possible public through English.

Recited Sanskrit—like the Latin of the Tridentine Mass—has an awesome and mysterious quality. A language could hardly be developed and used as an incantatory tool for three millennia without acquiring some kind of phonetic potency. The magic syllables of the 'perfect' language were treated as revelation, essential in helping the high gods to keep the demons at bay and maintain the *dharma* or proper order of things. Sanskrit is not, however, inherently superior to other languages, whatever gurus may say to the contrary. You can chant *om* or you can chant 'one'—which is a clearer focus for users of English than the great mystic syllable of Hinduism and Buddhism. Those, however, who like a bit of High Church ritual, as it were, will prefer *om* as their focusing agent.

Western science will probably, some day soon, come to terms with the physical and psychological effects of sounds vibrating in the human vocal tract. When that day comes, I suspect it will in fair measure be due to investigation of the voice technology of brahmin and guru. It will in the process demonstrate that Sanskrit is well shaped for incantation, but not that it is the sole legitimate vehicle for mantras.

Sanskrit is pretty uniform throughout India, but there are inevitable variations in its use. North Indians, for example, speak languages that are in the main historically linked with Sanskrit, much as Italian is historically linked with classical Latin. When present-day North Indians use Sanskrit, therefore, they adapt it to their own languages even when they use the words in English, just as Italians have adapted Latin. The general effect is shown in the following table:

Traditional Sanskrit terms	*Modern North Indian Sanskrit terms*
Rama	Ram
Veda	Ved
asana	asan
Gautama Buddha	Gautam Buddh
jnana	gyan
karma-yoga	karam-jog
yantra-mantra	jantar-mantar
samsara	sangsar

South Indians, on the other hand, speak languages that do not have a historical link with Sanskrit, although Sanskrit words have poured into their languages just as Latin has poured into English. As a result, Sanskrit expressions in a language like Tamil stand out just as Latin phrases like *ipso facto* and *ignis fatuus* stand out in a text of English. South Indians tend also to present Sanskrit words in their English in slightly fuller forms, so that *mantra* for them is *mantram*, and *darshana* is *darshanam*. But none of these variations, northern or southern, affects the meanings of the words in any way whatsoever.

The same is true of the peculiar effect that the British at large have had on Sanskrit and other Indian words from the late eighteenth century onward. Britons used a rough-and-ready approach when re-spelling Sanskrit into English, producing oddly homely-looking words with a touch of humour about them that is sometimes amiable and sometimes condescending. A typical early example was the adaptation of the name of the ruler of Bengal who was responsible in 1756 for the incident called the Black Hole of Calcutta. He was a Muslim called Siraj-ud-Dawlah whom the British re-named 'Sir Roger Dowler'—presumably a more manageable chap.

What can be called the Raj school of orthography has been on the wane since the Second World War, but its influence can still be found in older books on India and yoga and crops up in the names of people, shops, businesses, etc., in India, Mauritius and elsewhere even today. A fairly typical sentence in this style might be, 'Pundit Ramdass spoke to some Hindoos and Parsees about the Geeta', and the style can be tabulated as follows:

'British Raj' spelling	*'Indian Indian' spelling*
pundit	pandit
juggernaut	Jagannath(a)
Cawnpore	Kanpur
Bengalee	Bengali
Hindoostanee	Hindustani
kundalinee	kundalini

The biggest headache, however, comes with the academic transfer (or 'transliteration') of devanagari script into roman. All sorts of acute accents, bars, and dots are used for excellent scholarly reasons that are of no great value to the general reading public. Scholars need to be precise; for them the difference in the quality of a vowel or a consonant can be, for their purposes, as crucial as it was for the brahmins. Most people, however, are not academics, and their concern is easy use and recognition. It is also well established that languages which use a lot of these so-called 'diacritical marks' in their everyday scripts present their users with problems—'Have I dotted all my i's and crossed all my t's?' They can be tedious. A famous and little-loved diacritical mark in English is the apostrophe, and we know how badly it fares.

Unless a book, therefore, is by an academic for academics (and a limited public of people willing to make the special effort involved), in my own view the diacriticals are unnecessary and counter-productive. There are also variations among the systems used by scholars, which only add to the problem, although nowadays the transliteration of Sanskrit has been largely standardized. For those who have an interest in such matters, there are six main areas in which Sanskrit represented in roman script can pose problems:

1. s, ś, and ṣ

The first of these is the English 's', the second is the English 'sh', and the third is something like the 'ch' in the German *milch*. In effect, however, the two marked forms are adequately handled by 'sh', which is what I have done in this book, except when quoting.

2. ṛ

In Sanskrit this sound was a vowel, but in both English and the modern Indian languages this subtlety has little meaning. It can therefore be written as 'ri', so that the academic's *Ṛg-veda* can be everybody else's *Rig-veda*.

3. v and w

Most Indians pronounce these more or less like the English 'w', but few people are likely to change *Veda* to 'Weda' or, in the opposite direction, to turn *swami* into 'svami'. Expect a kind of 'w' from Indian speakers, but otherwise soldier on with the rather inconsistent usage that has established itself.

4. jn and c

The first of these is thoroughly misleading for most people and ought never to have been used in the first place. It should be pronounced as if the 'j' were the 'g' in *gun*, and *jnana* should be said like a nasalized *gyana*. The second item is pronounced like the 'ch' in *cheese*, so that *cakra* is indeed the same as *chakra*.

5. ṇ and ṁ or ṃ

By and large, this sound is the *anusvara* (or *anuswara*), a fully nasal consonant more like French than English. Words like *saṁsara/saṃsara* and *sannyasa* are nasalized in this way, but marking them can be tedious and not very useful, and is of scholarly interest only. Additionally, books differ, as for example between *Saṁkhya* and *Saṇkhya*. The scholarly form of 'Sanskrit' is *saṁskṛta*, and I am glad that we see it so rarely.

6. bh, dh, gh, kh, th

These are aspirated consonants; that is, a little puff of breath follows each 'b', 'd', etc. This is not a problem for English speakers, who do the right thing every day in words like 'clubhouse', 'madhouse', 'doghouse', 'bunkhouse', and 'hothouse'. If you find it awkward, however, there is no need to bother (although see below for *th*).

There are areas, however, where care is important. The first of these relates to stressed syllables, which correspond roughly in English to the long vowels of Sanskrit. Scholars usually put a flat bar (a macron) on top of these vowels, as in *āsana* and *prāṇāyāma*. Where Sanskrit has a long vowel, English has a stress or accent. Thus, the word *asana* is stressed on the first syllable, and not the second (as is often supposed); similarly, with *ananda*, *darshana*, *samsara* but the reverse for *Gautama*, *nirvana*, and *kaivalya*. Generally, *Upanishad* and *Arjuna* are stressed on the first syllable, while *pranayama*, *Mahayana*, and *yogasana* are stressed on the second. One simply gets used to it eventually.

The second area worth some attention is the pronunciation of 'th'. It is an aspirated *t*, not the 'th' in 'three' and 'thirty'. English comes closest to it in words like *guesthouse*. Pronouncing *hatha-yoga* as if it were normal English is a bit like pronouncing the 'ch' in 'chasm' as if it were the 'ch' in 'church'. Think *hatta*.

A word of warning to those speakers of English whose accent is Received Pronunciation or so-called BBC English. In Sanskrit the difference between the pronunciations and meanings of *kama* and *karma* are profound. No Indian could possibly confuse them, but in Received Pronunciation *karma-yoga* and the *Kama-Sutra* tend to sound as though they share the same first word. Some attempt should be made to distinguish them, preferably by giving *kama* ('desire') the 'a' of 'damn', while *karma* ('action') can have the 'a' in 'father'.

Another awkward area for Westerners is the Sanskrit talent for making compounds that look like one long word (not unlike German in this regard). Thus, *bhujangasana* is intimidating to eye and ear, but breaks readily enough up into *bhuja*, then *anga*, then *asana*: 'curve-body-position'. Since *bhujanga* can also mean a snake or cobra, that position is also often known quite simply as the Cobra. Similarly, *sarvangasana* divides up into *sarva*, *anga* and *asana*: 'whole-body-position'. Since it also happens to be a special kind of inverted pose, it is more commonly known as the Shoulder Stand, which does not translate it at all. Actual and potential teachers of physical yoga should have some awareness of these facts, just as doctors, nurses, and therapists have to master their terminologies.

Lastly, but intriguingly, comes the issue of explaining the technical terms of Sanskrit and yoga to one's audience. Gurus are not always scholars of Sanskrit etymology—their interests are elsewhere. As a result, they pass on in their discourses and in their books explanations of words which have nothing to do with their verifiable histories but a great deal to do with their mystical significance. This is entirely legitimate, but it can be confusing, because the special symbolism is presented as if it were etymology.

One example is the word *guru*. Its attested basic meaning is 'heavy' or 'weighty', implying 'important' and 'venerable', from which it was long ago extended to mean 'teacher' or 'spiritual guide'. However, some teachers and spiritual guides regularly explain *guru* by saying that *gu* means 'darkness' and *ru* means 'light'; a guru is therefore somebody who leads his disciples from the darkness of ignorance to the light of knowledge. Another example is *hatha*, whose attested basic meaning is 'force', 'effort' or even 'violence', but whose homiletic meaning is that *ha* is the sun and *tha* is the moon. The name of the famous treatise, the *Hatha-yoga Pradipika* can therefore be translated either literally as 'light on the yoga of effort' or symbolically as 'the light beyond the sun and moon [of duality]'. We can call these two styles of explanation the historical etymology and the mystical etymology respectively of yoga words, and should be on guard about confusing them.

Explaining these factors relating to Sanskrit-in-English is an exercise in cultural comparison, and in demonstrating what happens when cultures meet and mix. This meeting and mixing has been going on now for some time. It gathered momentum at the end of the eighteenth century and is now a strong current. Inevitably, confusions arise. But they can be handled, as I hope this book will help to show.

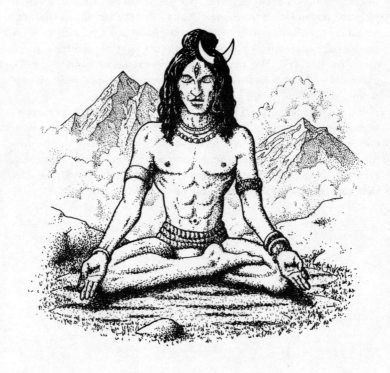

2. ASANA and YOGASANA

Kama the god of love was sent to waken Shiva out of the depths of meditation. It was a dangerous task, and Kama's reluctance was justified. The Great Yogi had retreated from the world, and would not take kindly to any being—god, human, or beast—that caused him to turn his attention outward again.

But the gods needed Shiva's help to destroy a tyrannical demon, and so little hesitant Kama had to persevere. He ascended Mount Kailas, and at its peak found the Great God seated on a tiger-skin, his legs crossed under him, his eyes closed, and his hands resting on his thighs, as calm and aloof as an ocean undisturbed by any ripple. The winds of the mountains did not dare come close, and the leaves of the trees were still.

Kama, however, disturbed that stillness by shooting a single arrow of desire into the Mahayogi, reminding Shiva of his lost love, the goddess Parvati. The hermit god stirred, and woke from his samadhi like a sea shaken by a sudden squall. Kama had done what he had been told to do, but he paid dearly for it. When Shiva saw who had disturbed him, he opened the third eye in his forehead and burned the god of desire to ashes.

This fragment from the ancient tale of Shiva's cosmic romance is replete with symbolism: the mountain-top of isolation, the calm ocean of inner peace, the sharp arrow of desire, and the third eye of enlightenment that alone can destroy desire. My main concern here, however, is not these images, important as they are, but the master image of the excerpt—a hermit seated alone in a remote place, wrapt in meditation like a cloak, withdrawn from the world of the senses and directed within.

That is the primordial image of *asana*.

The Sanskrit verb *as* means 'to sit', with connotations of dwelling, abiding, steadiness, and self-dedication. The noun *asana* derives from it, and can be glossed by such English words as 'sitting', 'a sitting posture',

or 'a seat', among others. In the *Bhagavad-Gita*, one of the classic texts
of yoga, the word *asana* is almost routinely translated as 'seat', so that a
reader of even three or four English-language versions of the *Gita* might
never know that the term had appeared in the original text at all. In the
Yoga-sutras of Patanjali, however, the reverse is the case; there, *asana* is
presented as a technical term, the third of the eight limbs of Patanjali's
Eight-Limb Yoga. In no English version of Patanjali is a reader likely to
escape a direct encounter with *asana*, either in Patanjali's aphorisms
themselves or in the various commentaries inserted between them.

Juan Mascaró's well-known translation of the *Gita* describes the yogi
seeking out 'a secret place, in deep solitude . . . a place that is pure and a
seat that is restful, neither too high nor too low, with sacred grass and a
skin and a cloth thereon. On that *seat* let him rest and practise Yoga for
the purification of the soul.'[2] *Asana* is the original of 'seat' in
both instances.

Swami Vivekananda's equally well-known translation of—and
commentary upon—the *Yoga-sutras* lists the eight limbs of Patanjali's
classical yoga as: Yama, Niyama, Asana, Pranayama, Pratyahara,
Dharana, Dhyana, and Samadhi. He further translates the aphorism on
asana as 'Posture is that which is firm and pleasant', adding the
commentary: 'Now comes Asana, posture. Until you can get a firm seat
you cannot practise the breathing and other exercises. Firmness of seat
means that you do not feel the body at all . . .' Later, he translates: 'Seat
being conquered, the dualities do not obstruct,' adding the information
that the dualities are such pairs of opposites as heat and cold, good and
evil, and so forth.[3] A good seated posture therefore assists the student to
overcome the confusions of the world.

The legend of Shiva, the recommendations of the *Gita*, and the
requirements of Patanjali are all in broad agreement about *asana*. They
represent traditions which date from the first millennium BC—well over
two thousand years ago—and their harmony on this point is reassuring;
but this harmony is different from the statements (and practices) of
many later exponents of yoga, all of whom—with due Hindu
deference—accept such early classics as the basic texts of their
discipline. It is not at all unusual for Hindus to blend and adapt different
traditions and ideas—Swami Vivekananda does this very elegantly, for
example, in his works—but the result can be confusing at times for the
Western student of the subject, and works in English are not always
entirely clear on the nature and evolution of the term *asana*.

The point at issue here is that the earliest sources do not divide *asana*
up into *asanas*.

Manipulating one's body for ascetic-mystical purposes is an ancient and respected activity in India. If, however, the compilers of the *Gita* and the *Yoga-sutras* engaged in bending, stretching, contracting, twisting, tensing, relaxing, and binding in various ways the whole or any part of their bodies in stylized poses, they say nothing at all about it. Given the importance that such poses have for so many people engaged in yoga, this is a matter of some interest.

In early yoga treatises, ascetic practices are grouped under the term *tapas*, literally translated as 'heat'. This was and is understood to be psychophysical energy generated by undertaking rigorous bodily and mental tests that bear some resemblance to the initiation rites and magical practices of many so-called 'primitive' people around the world. Appropriate *tapas* is advocated in both of the classics and figures as a sub-category of *niyama* in Patanjali. There it is often translated as 'austerity', and as Alain Daniélou puts it: 'Austerity burns all impurities and leads to the achievement of great mental and sensory powers.'[4]

The *Gita* distances itself from extreme forms of ascetic practice, recommending instead a moderate austerity, but at the same time it also uses the image of yoga burning away the dross of life. Neither work, however, directly links *tapas*—which remains largely undescribed—and *asana*, which is simply sitting.

For centuries however, forest hermits had imposed a prodigious variety of physical tests upon themselves that included such rigours as sitting or standing, or standing on one leg, or standing with one or both arms raised, for hours on end, as well as sitting and standing in hot places or in freezing water. Such activities were slowly systematized, coming in the early Middle Ages within the ambit of Tantra, a highly ritualized and magical form of Hinduism that became popular and powerful well after the writing down of the two classics just mentioned. In crude general terms, the Tantric seeker strove upwards from the taming of the body through the stilling of the mind to an understanding of that spirit which was perceived as both in each individual and behind the discernible cosmos. This was not a new idea—it is all already there in the classics—but the ways in which the Tantrics developed it were new, and included that development of yogic ideas called *hatha-yoga*.

Hatha means 'effort', 'force', and even 'violence'. Macdonell's *Sanskrit Dictionary* adds to its basic definition: 'forced meditation (a kind of Yoga attended with great self-torture)'. Its refinement took place during the Indian Middle Ages, towards the end of the first millennium AD, and is associated in particular with three sages: its founder Matsyendra (one of the 84 legendary *siddhas* or 'perfected ones'), Goraksha, and Swatmarama, who is credited with the authorship of the *Hatha-yoga Pradipika*. This is only one of the many hatha-yogic treatises that are not well known nowadays either inside or beyond India, but have had a more direct influence on shaping people's ideas of yoga than either the *Gita* or the *Yoga-sutras*. These treatises are the original models for the current manuals of 'physical yoga' available both in the East and the West.

It was in manuals like these that the detailed classification of many distinct *asanas*—indeed, of the *yogasanas*—first appeared. Of the manuals and the number and diversity of these poses, Daniélou says:

Of the theoretical eighty-four times one hundred thousand postures, eight-four only are generally known and specially important, and, of these, thirty-three only are said to give good results, and two only can be practised by anyone. Different asanas are described in detail in different books of yoga. The Hatha-yoga Pradipika describes 14, the Yoga Pradipa 21, the Gheranda Samhita 32, the Vishva Kosha 32, the Anubhava Prakasha 50. All however agree that the number of the chief postures is 84, although there exist some technical differences in defining them.[5]

As Georg Feuerstein puts it, in Tantra the body is not a hindrance to supreme enlightenment, but a temple of the divine: 'The primary intention of Hathayoga is to prepare the body for the higher spiritual practices, to "bake" it hard in the fires of physical Yoga . . . It purports to be a ladder to Rājayoga which emphasizes the virtue of meditative discipline.'[6]

Clearly, ideas varied among the hatha-yogis as to what exactly the asanas were and how many were useful. Equally clearly, for them the concept of *asana* had moved into a whole new area of speculation and experimentation. Their basic poses were still forms of sitting (the lotus, the hero, the adept, and the prosperity poses) but the other poses share with the concept of 'seat' only the goal of meditative calm. Apart from that, they draw upon *tapas* and upon the magico-religious tradition that the shamans of Siberia, the medicine men of old North America, the witch-doctors of Africa, and the voodoo priests of the Caribbean also share. It is, however, a tradition and a worldview for which Western science and education currently have little respect.

Benjamin Walker captures the magico-religious side of the hatha-yogic *asanas* when he observes:

Patanjali recommended a sitting position that was 'firm and agreeable', steady and comfortable. Attempts to meet this need have resulted in more than a thousand different postures, only three or four of which can really be said to fulfil the very modest requirements laid down. Many asanas are, as it were, plastic moulds assumed by the human body in the shape of some object, plant or animal, in the belief that the qualities that characterize that thing will imbue the yogi assuming it. There are asanas named after the lion, bull, camel, tortoise, swan, crane, locust, scorpion, tree, lotus, thunderbolt, bow, plough, and hundreds more.

Each brings its own benefit and is intended to approximate by sympathetic vibratory resonance to the object or animal concerned. Photographs of the contortions invented by the practitioners reveal their extraordinary ingenuity in trying to fit the human body into preconceived moulds of these various prototypes.[7]

Adopting ritual shapes and creating a geometry of mysticism is integral to Hindu culture, whether it is part of religious ceremony, art and decoration, dance-drama, or the meditative disciplines. The *mudra* ('gesture') is common to religion, dance, and yoga, while both *murtis*, the figures of deities, and the meditational diagrams called *yantras* depend upon the assumption that the same fundamental patterns repeat themselves throughout the universe—and everywhere have their quota of power. All such shapes and patterns are like the burning glass that focuses the power of the sun; concentrate upon them, or better still adopt them yourself, and you obtain a key to mastery over self and nature. In the microcosm of the body one can imitate the macrocosm of the world and tune in to it, part by part, nerve by nerve, centre by centre, until each element of the human being corresponds to—and vibrates and merges with—the proportionate part of the Cosmic Being.

That was the Tantric theory behind the work of the hatha-yogi. Starting with his own body and the physical world around him, he focused on what was immediately observable: nature in the form of animals, plants, weather, mountains, rivers, and so forth, with their geometry and their attributes, all aspects of the Great Being Shiva. Resemblance ritual became physical technology, the creative imitation of, and concentration upon, the virtues or essence of lions, crocodiles, lotuses, trees, swastika designs, gurus, weapons, and tools resulting in the *simhasana, makarasana, padmasana, vrikshasana, svastikasana, virasana/ siddhasana/Matsyendrasana, dhanurasana,* and *halasana* . . .

The lotus seat called *padmasana* derives from the nature of the lotus water lily as perceived through the Hindu eye: a delicate spreading spiritual beauty on a slender stem, floating on the water of life and rising from the mud below. Adopt the lotus pose with stylized, geometric perfection and you too will rise like the lotus from the mud of life and extend spiritual petals to the sun. The tree posture called *vrikshasana*, as B.K.S. Iyengar points out, 'tones the leg muscles and gives one a sense of balance and poise'[8], but only because it imitates and absorbs the strength and rooted balance of a tree. The yogi does not accidentally look like a lion when he performs *simhasana* with its formalized snarl; as

Daniélou puts it, he expects to be feared when he imitates the scorpion through the *vrishchikasana*.[9] When the spine is bent like a bow in the *dhanurasana*, the arrow of the spirit can be sent to its target, and when enough such *asanas* are perfected—along with the other techniques of hatha-yoga—the practitioner becomes the sum of all of them and moves through a range of powers until he becomes one, for ever, with the Great Yogi atop Mount Kailas, who can burn desire to ashes with one glance from the third eye of detachment.

Daniélou takes the idea of resemblance ritual a stage further when he brings in the Tantric picture of special psychophysical centres in the body that are known as the *chakras*. Referring to these as 'centres, or points where the gross and subtle bodies are joined', he states that such centres are grouped differently for different species:

Each living species is characterized by a difference in the relative positions of these centres and this can be represented by a geometrical figure. If we deliberately place the centres of the [human] body in a given relative position, creating the geometrical figure characteristic of a certain species, we enter into contact with the cosmic entity which manifests itself in that particular species. Many of the bodily postures are therefore associated with different beings or animals.[10]

Conventional Western thought cannot easily come to terms with theories and practices like these. It is far easier to re-adjust the lens of enthusiasm and see the *asanas* as simply techniques for toning up the body, giving one greater health and strength, promoting long life and an enviable tranquillity. If this then provides a better physical base for mental development and some kind of spiritual progress beyond that, so much the better. But becoming one with the lotus in its pond and acquiring the poise of a tree, or engaging in the psychic geometry of a lion . . .

The conceptions proposed here are not so much mystical as magical. Western occultists like Daniélou have no difficulty in adapting to them, or adapting them to Western occult tradition, but Western science and the average person curious about yoga have a harder time. People interested in scientific method usually see themselves as engaged in a long-drawn-out war with things like 'magic' and 'superstition', while the average person educated in the broad traditions of the West does not know what to think about such things as geometric symbolism, cosmic entities, and magical mimicry. The safest conclusion for many who have developed an interest in yoga is to suppose that the yogis may have started out with ideas like that, but, like the alchemists who slowly turned into chemists, found other and more practical benefits along the way.

This is a comforting and entirely legitimate approach to adopt. Most people involved with yoga would agree that the hatha-yogis and their predecessors acquired all sorts of practical experience of, and knowledge about, the body through their pursuit of magical and mystical goals. One area in which yoga and Western medical science can meet as equals is in the exploration of the physical gains and therapeutic potential of yogic exercise. While this is a great deal, however, it is not enough. Yoga is not just a system that can be taken in part into the Western medico-scientific bag of tricks. It is altogether too large and too significant for that. It must meet Western ideas on its own terms, part of which is its ancient magical aspect. That side of yogá requires from the West a caution, a respect, and a careful attention that have not yet been accorded to it. This is not to say that 'magic' must be accepted lock, stock and broomstick; but it does mean that the purposes and effects of magical usage need adequate study.

Science is part of the Western heritage, just as yoga is part of the heritage of the East. Even those Westerners who are enthusiastic about the occult and mysticism cannot reject science and rationalism entirely, any more than a Hindu with a rational and materialist bent can reject the magical yoga heritage; it is in the cultural air they have been breathing since childhood. At the same time, the dedicated Western or Westernized rationalist has to beware drawing rigid conclusions about theories and practices in very different civilizations on the basis of what contemporary science 'knows' to be true. Science also evolves and is at the end of the day just as limited an artifact of Western culture as yoga is a limited artifact of Eastern culture.

One Westerner who has attempted an analysis of magic was Sir James G. Frazer in *The Golden Bough* (1890). He saw it essentially as a pre-logical condition, pre-dating in our social evolution the religious stage which in turn pre-dates the scientific stage—for him the highest stage. Frazer's observations are appropriate here because they were seminal for future Western theories of culture and also because he coined the phrase 'sympathetic magic' for the kind of thing that the hatha-yogis were attempting, or that voodoo priests attempt in other ways. If you concentrate enough on an associative ritual, Frazer's 'savage' believed, then that ritual will affect the thing with which it is associated. Thus, a properly performed dance that simulates rain will stimulate rain; the eating of an enemy's heart will give you the bravery possessed by that enemy; drawing bison on a cave wall in natural colours will give you power over those bison in real life when you go to hunt them. Or, take up the lotus pose and you will become like the lotus. Metaphor is not just saying that x is like y, but that x is—or can be—exactly what y is.

Frazer's 'sympathetic magic' and Walker's 'sympathetic vibratory resonance' are not very far apart except that Walker proposes some kind of energy correspondence between yogi and imitated object that Frazer would never have tolerated. Frazer wholly disbelieved in associative ritual, which he saw as a kind of false reasoning, and science knows nothing about 'good vibes' and 'bad vibes'. The ancient yogis, however, firmly believed in what they were doing, and did it assiduously. In the process, whatever else they developed, they discovered that the various *asanas* had important physical consequences: some were generally beneficial, some were dangerous, some were dangerous under certain circumstances but beneficial if managed with care, and so forth. The hatha-yogis were able to delay the onset of old age and have acquired quite marvellous ascendancy over not just their behaviour, their emotions, and their muscles, but even over the 'autonomic nervous system', that part of the body's controls which, in the view of the Western medical scientists who invented the phrase, could not respond to the promptings of the conscious mind. Hatha-yogis, unaware of this 'scientific' restriction, have done and continued to do things with their heartbeat, respiration, and metabolism that until recently were simply *impossible* as far as science was concerned. If science has now revised its understanding of the body and brain, it is in part due to the proof provided by the 'non-scientific' hatha-yogis.

Nowadays, the *asana* of the classics and the *asanas* of the hatha-yogis have been married in what looks at first like a successful union. The following comment by B.K.S. Iyengar sums the state of affairs up neatly:

The third limb of yoga is asana or posture. Asana brings steadiness, health and lightness of limb. A steady and pleasant posture produces mental equilibrium and prevents fickleness of mind. Asanas are not merely gymnastic exercises; they are postures. To perform them one needs a clean, airy place, a blanket and determination, while for other systems of physical training one needs large playing fields and costly equipment. Asanas can be done alone, as the limbs of the body provide the necessary weights and counter-weights. By practising them one develops agility, balance, endurance and great vitality.[11]

Three views of *asana* appear to be possible. Firstly, as described in the *Gita* and the *Yoga-sutras*, *asana* means 'seat', and this meaning is sufficient. Secondly, *asanas* are multifarious, ranging from the simplicity of the two yoga classics to the complexities of the hatha-yoga manuals. Thirdly, there are two distinct views of *asana*, an earlier simple one and a later complex one, and these two views are not easily reconciled.

We are free to choose the view that best suits us, or to appreciate that three views exist and keep our options open. The majority of people who are interested in yoga would probably go for the second option, along the lines of Iyengar's definition, but those who prefer the first view of *asana* need not feel disturbed by this; after all, they have the *Gita* and the *Yoga-sutras* on their side. I tend myself to incline towards the third position.

Georg Feuerstein takes the Iyengar view a little further when he looks at the intrinsic purpose and worth of *asana*. For him, it is 'not purely a physical exercise, although it is, today in the West, widely imitated as just that. The yogic posture is assumed with a definite inner disposition, of which full awareness and peace are the most outstanding components. By drawing in the dispersed members of the body and by uniting them so as to form a homogeneous whole, the *yogin* awakens the intrinsic aliveness of his body. This is the first stage in the actual process of directing the consciousness inwards.'[12]

Iyengar also insists that the *asanas* are no more than a preparation; they are not ends in themselves, as responsible exponents of the craft usually take pains to point out. Feuerstein has gone a little further, however, by suggesting that Western imitation of yogic postures is often 'a purely physical exercise'. This kind of imitation is not, apparently, as sound as the yogis' imitation of their target animals, plants, natural objects, ideas, and sages. The implication is that the sanitized and packaged courses offered in Europe and North America may be based on yoga, may echo yoga, but are not actually instilling yoga itself. The inner dynamic, he hints, is missing.

Perhaps it is, in some quarters. It is equally possible, however, that certain adapters of yoga do not want—or do not perceive themselves as needing—that particular inner dynamic. The associative geometric magic may simply be meaningless to them, whereas the benefits to the cardio-vascular system, the glands, and the muscles may be apparent and real. They are not only free to adapt yoga in the direction of strictly physical and psychological therapy or training, but may well achieve a greal deal by doing so. Further, it is always possible that while concentrating 'imitatively' on the forms, they may acquire, through the 'magic' of successful and regular imitation, an increasing awareness of those other non-physical dimensions in which yogis in India have always been interested.

There would appear to be room for everybody; certainly, no board of censors has ever existed or is ever likely to exist which delimits the subject and says that only certain practices and concepts are to belong within the ambit of 'yoga'. The complex tradition embodied in this one word appears to be capable of adaptation and extension in all sorts of ways, only one of which is a physical-fitness orientation in the West.

Deploring such an orientation is unlikely to make it go away, and its departure if it did go away would surely be regrettable, as it could provide some very useful services indeed in the broad area of fitness, health, and psycho-physical therapy.

At the same time it is unwise to suppose, as some people do, that physical manipulation is the only preparatory technique for yoga. The simpler interpretation of *asana* in the early classics—that it is 'seat' and no more than that—makes this point clear. To be interested in the wider aspects of yoga, and in the ultimately non-physical goals of the subject, people do not need to follow a regime of bodily activities. From this point of view the *asanas*—however interesting, however physically and psychologically useful in themselves, however challenging—are only one avenue via which yoga may be initially explored.

Many disciplinary techniques are possible through which one can focus the personality and work towards some sort of personal integration. In India, parallel techniques include the chanting of mantras and the drawing and visualizing of yantras, as well as meditating upon the *murti* or form of a deity. Following an occupation or developing a craft to its highest point have also been recommended; selfless service, devotional behaviour, and intellectual effort offer additional or distinct paths on the way to concentrating body and mind so as to appreciate what they are and what lies beyond them.

Focus and concentration are the central issues in yoga rather than the specific techniques and devices used in focusing and concentrating.

3. Ashram and Ashrama

The ashram consisted of a group of low, white-washed huts in a grove of spreading trees. Below the compound is the river in which women pound their laundry on the flat stones and cows and buffaloes wade. All around, the scene is gently pastoral but near by are twisted masses of closely packed slum dwellings huddling under the ugly smokestacks of the Ahmedabad textile factories whose owners financed the ashram. Gandhi's room was about the size of a cell; its window had iron bars put there by a former occupant. Except for intervals in prison, Gandhi lived in that cell for sixteen years.

Some of the most active leaders of the independence movement began their political careers at the feet of the Mahatma at Sabarmati. The population of the settlement fluctuated from 30 at the start to 230 at its maximum. They tended the fruit trees, spun, wove, planted grain, prayed, studied, and taught in the surrounding villages. An air of soft repose and tranquillity still hovered over the ashram when I visited it in 1948, a decade and a half after Gandhi had moved elsewhere.[13]

So wrote the American journalist and author Louis Fischer in 1954, describing not some ancient, myth-suffused shrine, but a powerhouse of the spirit in which a modern karma-yogi presided as his spinning-wheel over the liquidation of the British Indian Empire. The description is as paradoxical as one could possibly hope for in a land renowned for paradox: the gathering-place of the voluntarily poor has been financed by the inordinately rich; pastoral scenes co-occur with the dark satanic mills and slums of industrialization; a man who has retreated from the world trains men who will change that world; an ashram cell is indistinguishable from a prison cell, and yet its owner is freer in both than most other people in the finest of houses.

A few lines earlier, Fischer has made his own comments on the traditional spiritual centres of India: 'In ancient India, ashrams were religious retreats for monks. Ashramites resigned from the world, and contemplating themselves inside and out, waited for the end. Gandhi's ashram, however, remained in closest contact with the world. In fact it

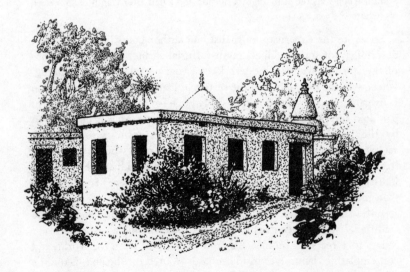

became the navel of India. Indians contemplated it and began a new life.'

Fischer's is a fairly typical Westerner's observation of such things, and is not without a share of truth: much of Hindu and Buddhist tradition has been world-denying, while India is in all likelihood the place of origin of every kind of monasticism, Eastern or Western. But Fischer's is not a complete vision, because Mohandas Karamchand Gandhi, however innovative, was in many ways a Hindu conservative and in establishing his ashram did not necessarily suppose for one moment that withdrawing from the world meant giving up all influence over that world. Quite the contrary, in fact: there is a tradition that is as old as monasticism itself, which maintains that 'monks' are as necessary to the world as soldiers, sailors, steel-makers, merchants, and farmers, perhaps more necessary, because the vocation is so demanding.

In fact, the curious paradoxical problem of simultaneous retreat and involvement is contained in the Sanskrit word *ashrama* from which 'ashram' comes, because it has two meanings that appear not to fit together at all.

At first sight there is nothing complicated about the idea contained in the now thoroughly English word 'ashram'. As one up-to-the-minute dictionary puts it: 'the hermitage of a Hindu wise man; broadly, any Hindu religious retreat'.[14] People generally and rightly think of a settlement centred upon a guru of importance. That guru might have started the ashram deliberately, or might simply not have prevented it from starting; indeed, ashrams from time to time simply grow up in the shadow of the guru.

Because of both the Gandhian connection and hippie-cum-socialist influences, ashrams are often conceived as utopian communes, a collectivity pervaded by the authority of the one who justifies its existence. Members come and go, while a core of the truly devoted resides there permanently, and all believers share in the *darshana* or radiating presence of the god-like teacher. Work and even property may be shared, and the place may even retain its power, as Fischer's words suggest, when the guru has abandoned it.

It is therefore both an escape from the world, and a model for the world to follow—or so the faithful believe. It may even be proclaimed as a foreshadowing of life in a New World just dawning.

The idea of a model for living is central to the other meaning of *ashrama*, which appears to date from the tensions that arose 2,500 years ago when Gautama the Buddha and other philosophical radicals offered alternatives to the leadership of the brahmins. For centuries, since the Aryans arrived in the sub-continent, the brahmin caste had been establishing itself as a god-like élite. Their sacrifical rituals, they maintained, helped the higher gods to govern the universe, while their guidance to other mortals provided the only gateway to self-improvement on this earth and elsewhere. The brahmins were the keepers of the sacred Vedas, were custodians of the holy language called Sanskrit, and constantly justified the vast and complex institution nowadays called the caste system.

They did not have complete mastery, however, over thought and action in ancient India, and for two reasons. Firstly, the Aryans had imposed themselves on a pre-existing Dravidian population with its own cultures, cities, languages, ideas, and cults: these did not simply go away, but had to be assessed, and resisted or absorbed. Secondly, the kshatriya caste—the warriors and governors among the Aryan clans—did not meekly accept the claims of the priests to be the highest caste, and legends and philosophical works, in particular the *Upanishads*, are full of indications that the warriors had their own alternative tradition. In addition, the kshatriyas mingled their blood-lines with the warrior-princes of the earlier stock, acquired many of their ideas, and—among other things—yoga appears to be one of the results of this blend. Yoga is a hybrid system of ancient Dravidian and more recently arrived Aryan, as indeed is much of popular Hinduism today.

The kshatriyas not only resisted the claims and ideas of the brahmins, but produced radical thinkers of their own who disputed these claims and ideas and finally rejected or bypassed the Vedas entirely. Along with the Vedas, they also bypassed the essential foundations of the caste system and offered systems of salvation that did not require brahmins at all.

The leading radicals were contemporaries from the area of Bihar in north-eastern India. They were Mahavira, the systematizer of Jainism, and Gautama, the creator of Buddhism, which have ever since been categorized by the brahmins as *nastika*—unorthodox doctrines. Both were ascetics, but Mahavira was extreme where Gautama was a relative moderate in such matters. They both rejected sacrificial offerings and ritual and denied the need for priests. Worse, they sidestepped the question of whether the gods were important and offered India tough-minded systems of self-help, making every individual on earth responsible for his or her own salvation. Those who defended the *dharma* or proper order in the universe, society, and each individual were inevitably anxious about this revolution. Before their eyes it was creating a new order of society in which humankind divided not into layered castes but into a mass of lay believers on one side and a novel élite of mendicant brethren on the other. This new order of beggar guides was non-productive and celibate and exalted non-productivity and celibacy over worldly work and the procreation of children. The world, they implied, was not worth having children in.

The orthodox counter-reformation was slow in developing, took centuries to gain momentum, but was eventually successful. By the middle of the first millennium AD it had reduced Jainism to a remnant and evicted Buddhism from its homeland, while largely reconciling brahmin and kshatriya. And one of the weapons in the spiritual armoury of resurgent Hinduism was the doctrine of the four *ashramas* or life stages.

Just as there were four great layered *varnas* or caste groups, so there were four stages through which a good caste-Hindu male should pass. These stages, applicable only to men of the top three castes (brahmin, kshatriya and vaishya), were as follows:

1. *brahmacharya* or celibate studenthood. When childhood was over, the young adolescent would be initiated into full status as a 'twice-born' Hindu, and should spend some years of austere study in the home of a chosen guru.

2. *grihastha*   Once well grounded in the Vedas, the young man would return to the family, marry, set up a household, beget children (especially sons), and fulfil his proper duties towards the gods, his ancestors, his caste, and society—including the charitable support of the right kind of holy men.

3. *vanaprastha*   When well into his later years, and having seen the birth of his children's children (especially grandsons), the house-holder should retreat into the forest to a hermit community, moving away from material things towards meditation and ascetic practices, including a relatively undemanding celibacy.

4. *sannyasa*   In age, the utter renunciation of the world, to become a *sannyasi(n)*, a wanderer without a home, who begs as he goes and prepares for death without ties of home or person, property or even caste.

In this life-plan, merit can be accumulated steadily by a proper adherence to convention, to the formalities, to order and to duty: there is a time and a place for everything that a right-minded man needs to do. Of this system, A.L. Basham says:

This scheme, of course, represents the ideal rather than the real. Most young men never passed through the first stage of life in the form laid down, while only a few went beyond the second. Many of the hermits and ascetics of ancient India were not old men, and had either shortened or omitted the stage of house-holder. The series of the four stages is evidently an idealization of the facts, and an artificial attempt to find room for the conflicting claims of study, family life and asceticism in a single lifetime. It is possible that the system of the *aśramas* was evolved partly as a counterblast to the unorthodox sects such as Buddhism and Jainism, which encouraged young men to take up asceticism and by-pass family life altogether, a practice which did not receive the approval of the orthodox, though in later times provision was made for it.

Despite their artificiality, however, the four stages of life were an ideal which many men in ancient India attempted to follow, and thus they deserve our consideration. Moreover they serve as a framework round which we can model the life of the individual.[15]

Although they were, like all model-making systems, an expression of the ideal as some person or group perceives it, and although like many other human endeavours they were only imperfectly followed and believed in, the four life-stages of brahminical Hinduism have never been revoked. Nothing in Hinduism ever *is* entirely revoked or superseded; everything simply accretes and blends in a vast, organic whole, at once a strength and a weakness. Because the idea is still there—especially in the traditions of the brahmins, who naturally applied their own rules more enthusiastically than the other upper castes—it is part of the luggage of the Hindu mind, and inevitably therefore part of the luggage of subjects like yoga.

Basham puts his finger on a key issue in Hinduism: that there is one tradition which insists that a man must fulfil his family and social obligations before he seeks his own salvation, and another quite contradictory tradition which insists that a true seeker after salvation and release will break with social obligation as soon as possible, sustain a totally celibate life, and renounce the world. Hindus swing between the extremes, as do numbers of Westerners who have been fascinated by Hindu spiritual life-styles. Swami Vivekananda speaks for the virtue of total renunciation in the following verse of his poem, *The Song of the Sannyasin*:

> They know not truth who dream such vacant dreams—
> As father, mother, children, wife, and friend.
> The sexless Self! whose father he? whose child?
> Whose friend, whose foe is He who is but One?
> The Self is all in all, none else exists;
> And thou art That, Sannyasin bold! Say—Om Tat Sat, Om![16]

This is the other sannyasin, not the aged wanderer of the four *ashramas*, but a man in his prime and a warrior of the spirit fighting a better fight than war, love, commerce, family, flesh, and the fevers of everyday existence. With masterly Hindu equivocation, however, Vivekananda can say elsewhere: 'The life of every individual, according to the Hindu scriptures, has its peculiar duties apart from what belongs in common to universal humanity. The Hindu begins life as a student; then he marries and becomes a householder; in old age he retires, and lastly he gives up the world and becomes a Sannyasin. To each of these stages of life certain duties are attached. No one of these stages is intrinsically superior to another. The life of the married man is quite as great as that of the celibate who has devoted himself to religious work.'17

In all probability Hindus have been so interested in transcending the paradoxes of life because their culture is so generously endowed with paradoxes. Certainly, this tension between total renunciation of the world and the flesh on the one side and concessions to a (properly ordered) world and flesh on the other side runs through much of Indian life and through many works on yoga. Take for example the following statement about *brahmacharya* by B.K.S. Iyengar:

According to the dictionary brahmacharya means the life of celibacy, religious study and self-restraint. It is thought that the loss of semen leads to death and its retention to life. By the preservation of semen the yogi's body develops a sweet smell. So long as it is retained, there is no fear of death. Hence the injunction that it should be preserved by concentrated effort of the mind. The concept of brahmacharya is not one of negation, forced austerity and prohibition. According to Śankaracharya, a brahmachari (one who observes brahmacharya) is a man who is engrossed in the study of the sacred Vedic lore, constantly moves in Brahman and knows that all exists is Brahman. In other words, one who sees divinity in all is a brahmachari. Patanjali, however, lays stress on continence of the body, speech and mind. This does not mean that the philosophy of Yoga is meant only for celibates. Brahmacharya has little to do with whether one is a bachelor or married and living the life of a householder. One has to translate the higher aspects of Brahmacharya in one's daily living. It is not necessary for one's salvation to stay unmarried and without a house. On the contrary, all the smṛtis (codes of law) recommend marriage. Without experiencing human love and happiness, it is not possible to know divine love. Almost all the yogis and sages of old in India were married men with families of their own. They did not shirk their social or moral responsibilities.18

Iyengar's closing statement is true; there is ample proof that the ancient yogic sages were married men. Unfortunately, his closing statement in this excerpt is also tranquilly at odds with his opening remarks about celibacy and semen, which in their turn harmonize with the following from Swami Vivekananda:

The Yogis claim that of all the energies that are in the human body the highest is what they call 'Ojas'. Now this Ojas is stored in the brain, and the more Ojas is in a man's head, the more powerful he is, the more intellectual, the more spiritually strong . . . Now in every man there is more or less of this Ojas stored up. All the forces that are working in the body in their highest become Ojas. You must remember that it is only a question of transformation . . . The Yogis say that that part of the human energy which is expressed as sex energy, in sexual thought, when checked and controlled, easily becomes changed into Ojas . . . [The Yogi] tries to take up all this sexual energy and convert it into Ojas. It is only the chaste man or woman who can make the Ojas rise and store it in the brain; that is why chastity has always been considered the highest virtue. A man feels that if he is unchaste, spirituality goes away, he loses mental vigour and moral stamina. That is why in all the religious orders in the world which have produced spiritual giants you will always find absolute chastity insisted upon. That is why the monks came into existence, giving up marriage. There must be perfect chastity in thought, word, and deed.[19]

Swami Vivekananda appears to be speaking for and about all yogis here, which is not really the case: yoga is a vast and tangled skein, and not everyone within that skein agrees about this important issue. However, many leading exponents of one or another kind of yoga tend to equivocate and blur this issue. Both Vivekananda and Iyengar do so here, but no one—however keen on equivocation—can deny that a particular yogic theory exists in which seminal retention (traditionally without discussing any female equivalent) is a vital factor. It is conceived less as moral continence than as part of a crucial alchemy of body, mind, and spirit that—whatever lip service is paid to the life of the householder—exerts an enormous psychological pull upon Hindu men who are interested in the mystical life. That it has also interested Westerners can be seen from the following, from Ernest Wood's *Yoga*:

. . . [Semen] draws its material from all over, and transmits something from every part of the body to the succeeding generation, and . . . waste of this fluid, or excessive generation of it, depletes the body all over, and on the other hand conservation of it is highly beneficial to the whole body. It appears that this is the one function of the body which does not work for the benefit of the body, but draws from it for the sake of another or others, and therefore its non-use does not harm the body but on the contrary is beneficial to it. This is at the back of the universal belief of the yogis in favour of continence and celibacy.[20]

Hindu and Hindu-derived theories and practice regarding sex, chastity, semen, and the idea of an alchemical transformation within the body are extremely complex. Thus, within especially Tantric cults that emerged in both Hinduism and Buddhism in the first millennium AD, strict chastity could be paralleled by special direct uses and sublimations of sexual intercourse. Geoffrey Parrinder, in his analysis of the sexual aspect of the world's religions, points to the significance in Hinduism of *coitus reservatus*. To hasten the rise of transmuted energy—the *kundalini* serpent—from the area of the genitals to the top of the head, partners in Tantric sex acts could will their sexual juices (more obviously in the man's case) to stay within the body, or, if ejaculated, to return to their source and in a mystic transubstantiation ascend the spine.

In certain kinds of Mahayana Buddhism, the practitioner could meditate upon the Vajra-Yogini ('the thunderbolt female yogi') and in so doing create an inner psychic heat:

The letter HAM, the Tibetan personal pronoun 'I', was to be visualized as white in colour like the semen which was thus set in activity. The goddess Kundalini, the serpent power, rose from her slumber below the navel to union with her lord in the highest centre of the skull. The symbolism was of phallic erection but retention of the semen or 'moon-fluid', which was transmuted into psycho-physical power. The aim, as in other sexual exercises of similar nature, was not ejaculation but transmutation of physical energy into spiritual and thereby attainment of salvation.[21]

A peculiar sexism pervades this whole aspect of India and yoga, the whole wrestling match between retreat to the ashram or life in the world, between total renunciation and chastity throughout life and planned renunciation at only certain stages in life. The nods towards 'the life of the householder' are also significant, because it is here that the female factor enters the equation. Largely, the discussion of yoga and the quest for spiritual power is couched in *male* terms, even if now and then it is briefly conceded that women are also included. The mainstream of traditional yoga is male, as is made clear by many references—those that I have quoted and others—to the importance of seminal fluid and its retention. Women are peripheral: they are distracting influences, have no real independence, and symbolize the risky snares of the world, a point which from time to time embarrasses exponents and describers of yoga who find themselves (in the West at least) addressing audiences mainly of women.

What I have just said is not universally true; there are aspects of yoga where women are by and large equal, and even occasionally in the ascendant. But it is largely true. The fundamental issue in both meanings of *ashrama* is what *men* should do with their lives in order to transcend worldly desire—whether or not they should scatter their seed in the wombs of women, or should hold on to it (self-fully if not simply selfishly) for their own private good. In the vocabulary and symbolism used, especially in the mystical process of raising the snake called *kundalini*, there is a nagging implication of spiritualized masturbation.

True potency, such practices imply, lies elsewhere, not in the life of the householder and his wife or wives. There is a contempt for both woman and the world, which are in any case blended, woman being the world and the creative illusion of *maya* being seen as female. Ascetics, while still manifestly virile, restrain, retain, and re-train their sexuality for a private orgasm of the soul. Such a man is the true hero, the *vira*, a word that is not too distant a cousin to the Latin *vir*, from which 'virility' derives.

The two *ashramas* meet in this question of sexual performance and abstinence, because the basic Sanskrit means 'religious effort'. One goes to an ashram as a retreat where one can engage in religious effort, while—ideally at least—a man practises the four *ashramas* as life-long religious effort. The argument, at its sharpest beween Buddhists and brahmins when the split first occurred, was whether true religious effort could be undertaken in a world where sexuality was an obligation.

Once, some years ago now, my wife and I spent some weeks on Mount Abu, a harshly beautiful volcanic cone that rises out of the Rajasthan desert in north-western India and a sanctuary over the centuries for holy men—and women. There are many temples and ashrams around the crater lake at the summit of the mountain, both Hindu and Jain. It is not permitted to kill any animals there, and everywhere in the little town centre or out across the hillsides one could come across naked sadhus, ash-covered and unkempt, or dignified robed figures at the temples and ashram gates. Sannyasis rented small caves from the Mahant of the Raghunathji Math, and *AUM* and other mantric graffiti could be found everywhere on the basalt rocks.

We visited a number of different religious groups on Abu, including the ashram of the Brahmakumaris or 'Daughters of God'. The aim of their movement was writ large on a notice by their gate: 'To reinherit Satyugi and Tretayugi viceless deity world sovereignty of 100 per cent Purity, Peace, Health, Wealth and Happiness for twenty-one generations which is yours most Beloved World's God-Fatherly Birthright. BUT BEWARE you can do so before destruction of this present Kalyugi vicious devil world.'

As we examined that rather startling announcement, a Hindu gentleman invited us into the ashram, where women with long loose hair and in white saris flitted about their work. We were hospitably served tea in a little room and were told that the ashram had been founded by Pitashree, a Sindhi who was the *avatar* or incarnation of Brahma. Whence the name Brahmakumaris, which could also be translated as 'Daughters of Adam', equating—as they did—the Hindu god Brahma with both the Judaeo-Christian Adam and the first saviour of the Jains, the primordial Adinath. We were told over tea that all history is a cycle of four ages, and that precisely 5,000 years ago this very same being Pitashree-Brahma started the cycle that is now drawing painfully to its close in the dissolute and destructive fourth age, Kali-yuga.

Pitashree was Shiva's representative on earth, inaugurator of a new golden age once this vicious devil world has been blasted apart by the nuclear weapons of the USA and the USSR. We were invited to affiliate ourselves to the ashram by both the gentleman and one of the ladies in white. It would not, they said, be necessary to give up the forms of everyday life. We could continue to live together as husband and wife, with only one proviso: there should be no further sexual contact and therefore no children.

We were both in our twenties at the time and had no children, although we now have three who are nearly adults and are getting ready to face the devilry of the world as best they can. My wife Feri was at the time amazed and amused by the Brahmakumaris, their offer, and the demand they made of total strangers hardly across their doorstep. She suggested afterwards in our hotel by Abu's crater lake that the Brahmakumaris' policy could be the answer to India's family-planning problem, and did not wish to pursue their acquaintance any further.

In order to hear Pitashree for myself, however, I returned as invited early the following morning and sat at his feet in the ashram. He was a man whose charisma did not reach me, but I listened and watched with interest, although his discourse was in Hindi and English interspersed and therefore hard to follow. The negation of the world was, however, amply expressed in not one but *three* vicious devil tape-recorders that were preserving his speech for imminent destruction.

The Brahmakumaris—who are also known as the Raja-yogis of Abu—are not far removed in spirit and style from the Jehovah's Witnesses, who also expect a terrible end to this terrible world, and imminently. In their white-walled ashram and their call to universal celibacy before it is too late, both for renunciants and for householders, they underline the permanent and unresolved tension among Hindus between the spiritual and the sexual.

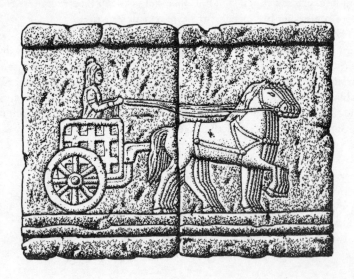

4. ATMAN and BRAHMAN

The *Maitri Upanishad* tells how King Brihadratha abdicated his throne in favour of his son and went alone into the forest. He had grown aware of the passage of time and the transience of the body, and had become indifferent to the things of this world. In the forest he became an ascetic, standing for hours with his arms raised, staring into the eye of the sun.

At the end of a thousand days the master Shakayanya came to him like the glow of a smokeless fire, and said:

'You have earned a boon. Name it.'

The royal ascetic bowed before his visitor, and said:

'Master, I am ignorant. Teach me about the *atman*.'

'That is a hard thing to teach,' said Shakayanya. 'Son of Ikshvaku, choose something else.'

The king fell to the ground and touched his head on the feet of his visitor, and said:

'Master, in this ill-smelling and insubstantial body, this collection of bone, skin, muscle, marrow, flesh, semen, blood, mucus, tears, rheum, excrement, urine, wind, bile and phlegm, what value is there in any other boon? In this body, assailed by desire, anger, greed, delusion, fear, despondency, envy, loss of the desirable, union with the undesirable, hunger, thirst, old age, death, disease, and grief, what else can be more worth knowing?

'Everything decays as we watch. Insects, plants and mighty trees all perish, as do such great warrior-kings as Sudyumna and Bharata, abandoning their people and their wealth alike. Even the gods and anti-gods die, oceans dry up, mountains crumble, the earth shakes and the stars tremble in the sky. The cycles of the ages turn—birth and death, re-birth and re-death. In this wheel of life I am like a frog in a waterless well. Deliver me from it all, Master, because you alone are my way of escape.'

Shakayanya nodded and smiled.

'Great king,' he said, 'your boon is granted, and you will know what *atman* is. It is your own self.'

'My own self?'

'The one who moves and never moves. The body is a cart that trundles along, and men have asked who drives that cart. The answer is that the one who stands aloof drives that cart, drives every cart, but the carts don't know. He knows our bodies, but our bodies do not know him.

'In the beginning there was one, and the one created the many. In each he placed a sliver of himself, giving them life like a wind stirring leaves. To each he has given five reins, some horses, a chariot and a charioteer. The senses are the reins, the horses are the organs of action, the chariot is the body, and the charioteer is the mind. The whip is each personality in this world of *maya*. Goaded by its driver, the body goes round and round like a potter's wheel— but the *atman* does not go round and round, though it moves from body to body, stained neither by bright deeds nor dark deeds and forever covered by the veil of what is. Behind that veil it is fixed and abiding.'

So Shakayanya taught the king, as other sages teach other students in other *Upanishads*. The subject is always the nature of the *atman*, a word that can be translated equally appropriately as 'self' or as 'spirit' or as 'breath'. In Sanskrit and in Latin respectively, *atman* and *spiritus* derive from the idea of breathing, although over the centuries they have moved from a primordial 'breath-soul' to the concept of something indestructible that is beyond and distinct from matter. *Atman* is not entirely alien; it is distantly related to the German *atmen* ('to breathe') and to the Greek *atmós*, the air that we refer to in 'atmosphere'. That is why Shakayanya could refer to life entering all creation like a wind, and why the breath-*atman* of the individual could so easily in Hindu metaphysics be equated with the wind-*atman* of the world: individual air with the world's air, individual spirit with the world's spirit.

The ancient Hindus therefore both meant and did not mean air and wind when they talked about *atman*; they might have started out long ages earlier supposing that the breath-wind was life itself, but later breath and wind were simply analogies for something infinitely further removed, in a realm beyond the senses. *Atman* cannot be directly perceived, and is hard to conceive; it is an abstraction, an essence tied to the thought—or, more properly, the mystical vision—that there is a base or ground or substratum to the universe that is beyond words to describe and is the absolute, imperishable originator, sustainer and dissolver of everything we know. Hindus argue, equivocate, and part company on all sorts of things, but they seldom argue, equivocate, or part company on this idea.

Hindu philosopher-theologians do, however, argue about the relationship that this ultimate bears to the creation or *maya* within which we live and move. A number of schools of thought have emerged, but two have been particularly influential, and essentially their argument rests on the idea of numbers and depends on whether you prefer a cool, emotion-free cosmos or would like a warm and loving personal link with it.

The *Upanishads* are the origin of the cool vision of how things are. Out of their poetic and mystical teachings has emerged a doctrine known as *advaita*, whose main proponents were the south Indian philosophers Gaudapada in the seventh century and Shankaracharya in the eighth and ninth centuries, summing up the age-long speculation that began in the *Vedas* themselves. This is the school of *Vedanta* ('the end or goal of the *Vedas*').

Advaita translates as 'not-two-ness' or, more tidily, 'non-duality'. Its argument is that the personal *atman* is, as the *Upanishads* maintain, a piece of the seamless robe called *Brahman*. This idea is neatly caught in English by an '*atman*' with a small 'a' and *the Atman* with a capital 'A'. At the same time, but mysteriously, this *atman-Brahman* is not separate from the web of creation that it has woven. They are not two either. Some scholars have therefore concluded that *advaita* can be translated as 'monism': that is, 'not two' means 'one'. This, however, is risky, because, as Alain Daniélou puts it: 'A Supreme Cause has to be beyond number, otherwise Number would be the First Cause. But the number one, although it has peculiar properties, is a number like two, three, or four, or ten, or a million. If "God" is one, he is not beyond number any more than if he is two or three or ten or a million.'[22]

In other words, we limit the ultimate when we say it is one, and the ultimate cannot be limited. It is therefore safer, in the view of the advaitists, to define the ultimate negatively, by saying *neti-neti* ('it is not this, not that') or by calling it non-dual, which is another way of saying that it is non-multiple.

This raises problems, however, because of the clear multiplicity of creation. As a consequence, an alternative interpretation grew up, also initially in south India, whose foremost philosopher was Ramanuja in the eleventh and twelfth centuries. His doctrine is known as *vishishtadvaita* or 'qualified non-duality': the ultimate is non-dual, but not quite the same as the creative web of *maya* that emanates from him. As a result, the myriad *atmans* that seek so insistently to return to the bosom of Brahman are justified in their desire, but the drop that returns to the shining sea of immensity is not dissolved utterly in that experience. Something of distinctness survives, allowing an awareness of worship and appreciation—indeed, of personality—and the Absolute in turn wishes such a distinction, indeed always planned for such a distinction, and is a personality too.

This is a much more theistic vision than the *atman-Brahman* equivalence of the *Upanishads*; it arose out of the devotion to the god Vishnu that surged up in south India and was one of the factors that contributed to the decline in its Indian homeland of the non-theistic Buddhist creed. Both Shankaracharya and Ramanuja were theistic brahmins, but they differed in their analyses and their emphases. Ramanuja was an enthusiast for the cult of *bhakti* or devotion that dated back at least to the *Bhagavad-Gita*, and saw it as the highest expression of the relation between creator and created. Shankaracharya accommodated such a view, but felt the need to transcend personalities and humanism, to transcend in effect any human-centred attribution to the Unlimited of human-like qualities. These were all right for the mass of believers perhaps, but they were not necessarily ultimate reality.

Shankaracharya's more clinical vision has remained of great significance to theorists, while Ramanuja's has been much more in tune with popular attitudes to deity and devotion. As A.L. Basham observes: 'Rāmānuja was not as brilliant a metaphysician as Śaṅkara, but Indian religion perhaps owes more to him than to his predecessor. In the centuries immediately following his death his ideas spread all over India, and were the starting-point of most of the devotional sects of later times.'[23]

Yoga has been influenced by both major views of the ultimate and its creation, being tinged in some cases by the idea of devotion to a personal god (as for example Krishna in the *Gita*), by a conception of an abstract 'lord' as a guide (the Ishvara of Patanjali's *Yoga-sutras*), by a similar conception of an elevated human guide (like Gautama the Buddha), or by a cool Vedantist conception of *atman* all unadorned with emotion and personality, where the droplet does indeed return to the shining sea, from which in fact it proves never to have been separate in the first place.

Such concepts, in the vigorous modern idiom, tend to blow the mind, and no doubt that was precisely what the sages have always wanted them to do. They illustrate once again the crucial problem of language: that words are not enough, that rational or even fantasy thought is not enough, that arguments will only get you so far and that myths and metaphors also only go part of the way. An appreciation of reality must by its very nature be beyond both vocalization and visualization, however useful these tools of our humanness are in getting us started on the journey. Eventually, inevitably, the road simply goes off all known maps . . .

Yet the rishis and the yogis of the past have always maintained that logical and metaphorical crutches *can* help; if not, no point at all to those forest dialogues in the *Upanishads* or the battle dialogue of Krishna and Arjuna in the *Gita*. As often as they used such images as breath and wind, they used the idea of language itself as an analogue for the ultimate, and it is in this usage that the word *Brahman* appears to have its origin. It is a dauntingly difficult word, but it cannot be glossed over or wished away.

Brahman as a word emerges from the world of the *Vedas*, where it was a prayer or sacred utterance, a verse, a text or a spell, so that it has something of the force found in the Gospel of St John: 'In the beginning was the Word, and the Word was with God, and the Word was God.' It extended to the whole sacred canon, to theology and learning, to the holy life, and to chastity (whence the related word *brahmacharya*). The people who possessed this *Brahman* in its most palpable form were, of course, the *brahmins*, whose actual Sanskrit name is a variant of the basic word. As the utterance behind the cosmos we come to *Brahman* as *Atman*, while within the sprawling cosmology of Hinduism at large there emerged a curious god-figure known as *Brahma*, who presides over an age that is a day of Brahma. He was yoked together in classical Hindu speculations with the rival gods Vishnu and Shiva to form the *trimurti*, the well-known trinity of Brahma the Creator, Vishnu the Preserver and Shiva the Destroyer of all things. Today, in India, *Brahm* is simply one possible name for 'God'.

Nothing is ever easy and straightforward in Hindu philosophy and cosmology, but what we *are* left with in this complex area is one of the most thrilling and chilling models of the universe that any culture has ever produced. That model can include 'God' as a personal and humane deity, single and imperishable, or can allow for a whole pantheon of hundreds of gods, super-gods and sub-gods, or can be essentially non-theistic, proposing a neutral ultimate 'it' that is there because it is there because it is there—and even 'it' is a useless pronoun with which to limit it. All images fail in the effort to describe the indescribable.

And that, like it or lump it, however described, is the target of yoga.

Yogis have never aimed at physical health and welfare for their own sake, nor mental balance and the stilling of the ripples of personality for their own sake. Whether they have taken up their tiger-skin and gone to sit on a mountain peak, or work daily in a city among rich and poor, sane and mad, black and white and brown, male and female, young and old, (all the polarities and variations of humanity), their aim has not been greater vitality, psychic powers, moderation in all things, or even the achievement of human perfection. These have all figured, and yoga did emerge out of both the warrior's and the priest's wish for naked power, but everything I have just listed is either a station along the way, or a bonus—a boon granted by a minor god, in passing.

The goal has always been to pierce the fog of existence, which is not always what one does two hours a week seated on the floor of the local school hall. It could be, but it usually isn't. Traditionally, it is not an enhancement of this life of bone, skin, and muscles, desire and delusion, but an abdication from it as a king gives up his throne to his eldest son and departs into the forest. That is a state of affairs whose implications many Westerners interested in yoga have yet to come to terms with.

5. AVATAR

In the *Bhagavad-Gita* Arjuna is the royal archer and Krishna is his charioteer. Standing between the two great armies drawn up for battle on the field of Kurukshetra, the chariot and its horses rest while Arjuna struggles with his duty and Krishna reminds him of that duty. Arjuna does not wish to take part in civil strife, when he will be forced to kill his kinsmen, his friends, and his teachers, but Krishna tells him that he must, tells him that action undertaken without a desire for reward carries no scars into the next life. In the process of urging Prince Arjuna on to battle in a just cause, Krishna imparts to him ancient secrets about yoga, and says of them, in Chapter 4:

'Once, long ago, I explained all this to Vivasvat, the sun. He told it to Manu, the first man, and Manu passed it on to Ikshvaku. So the tradition was handed down, and the royal seers learned it, the kingly rishis. But in course of time the yoga was lost. It is a great mystery, this ancient lore, and I am only telling it to you now because you are my loyal friend.'

Arjuna was wretched and bewildered, and said: 'You were born *later* than the sun. The sun was created long *before* you. What on earth do you mean by saying such things as "I explained this yoga long ago"?'

'Arjuna,' answered Krishna, driver of the chariot, 'I have had many births, and so have you—but I remember all of mine, and you remember none of yours. In my ultimate self, though, I am changeless and am never born at all—ever. I am the lord of all beings, and through my power of *maya* I blend with nature and take shape. Whenever the rightful *dharma* fails and anarchy appears I project myself in a form like this. I re-appear from age to age, for the protection of the good and the destruction of evil-doers, and to rebuild the social order. Anyone who comprehends that truth, Arjuna, escapes re-birth.'

Krishna does not call himself an *avatar*, but this is the great statement around which what Geoffrey Parrinder calls 'avatar theory' has crystallized. On the philosophical tensions at the time of the *Gita* and later, Parrinder says:

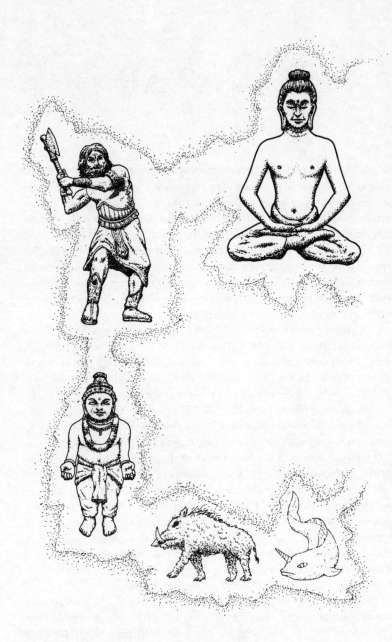

After other priestly texts the Vedas were followed by the Vedanta, the 'Veda's end', or Upanishads. This speculative religious philosophy probed into the nature of the neuter divinity, Brahman, and its relationship to the gods and the human soul. It arrived at the non-dualism (*advaita*), or monism, which later Vedantic philosophers like Śankara cherished as the quintessence of Upanishadic thought. The key verse, THAT THOU ART (*tat tvam asi*) identified the divine and the soul, and appeared to abolish any dualism or subject-object relationship between God and man.

For religious life, however, some kind of objective relationship with a deity seems to be necessary, and even the Upanishads began to show that, whatever might pass for philosophy, a monistic or a godless religion was not enough.[24]

In Hinduism there have been waves of gods, some of whom have waxed and waned, some dwindled to nothing, others come from minor status into awesome majesty, some from apparently nowhere to high status. Hindus regard the matter quite lightly: gods come and go too, just like mortals, but the great gods go on for ever, and behind the great gods is the truly great god . . . Thus, such gods of the *Vedas* as Varuna, Mithra, and Bhaga have vanished away or been transformed out of all recognition, while others like Indra remain as shadows of their former Olympian selves, continuing down the centuries as characters in morality plays rather than as high and seriously worshipped deities. From classical times onward, three major divinities have occupied centre stage, two of them conceived as male and one as female, and each the love-object of enormous 'sects'. These super-deities are Vishnu, whose followers are the Vaishnavas, Shiva, whose followers are the Shaivas, and a goddess of many names who is often known as Shakti, and whose followers are Shaktas.

For at least two thousand years these have been the true divine competitors for the hearts and minds of Hindus, pushing aside into the cells and hermitages of holy men the arguments about *atman* and *Brahman*—and fomenting discord as each group has pushed its own divinity forward as the god of gods, or the fullest manifestation of 'God'. The matter is further complicated by two historical trends: firstly, to see Vishnu as a whole host of lesser god-figures in one, and, secondly, to conceive Shiva and Shakti as a divine pair. Thus, the followers of Vishnu are spread out across a diversity of Krishna cults, Rama cults, and other groups, while the followers of Shiva and Shakti sometimes mingle as the followers of Shiva-Shakti. And finally, of course, no group denies the godhood of the god of any other group, only the pre-eminence of that deity.

However, before taking the issue of the *avatar* further, it makes sense to consider just how all of this relates to yoga. After all, one can proceed through quite an extensive course of poses (*asanas*), breath control (*pranayama*), locks (*bandhas*), and seals or gestures (*mudras*) without ever encountering the term or the idea. And there is nothing in the *Yoga-sutras* of Patanjali or the majority of the Upanishads about *avatars*. Even where the idea is strongly present in the *Gita*, the word itself is not used, while by and large it is true to say that one can make considerable advances in yoga without a commitment to any god or to God, or even the view that divinity exists. After all, yoga is akin to Buddhism, and Buddhists do not have gods as the centrepieces of their faith.

The reason for taking an interest in *avatars* is, I think, three-fold. Firstly, one understands yoga better if one understands its Hindu setting better. Hinduism and Buddhism are the matrices in which yoga developed over thousands of years, and it is only in the last few years that internationalized yoga has begun to reformulate itself in ways which are not specifically Hindu or Buddhist. If international Westernized yoga is a continuing and useful trend, which I think it is, then the more we know about the cradle of the subject the better. It may well help us see where we are going.

Secondly, although the word *avatar* is absent from the *Gita*, the idea is so fundamental to that classic treatise on the yogic life that to ignore it would falsify the evidence. In the *Gita*, Krishna is the ancient founder and teacher of yoga, a god descended to help humankind, and his advice throughout the work relates to yogic activity. In this he rivals the other god, Shiva, who is often called the Mahayogi ('the Great Yogi'). If one looks at the symbolism of Shiva to understand yoga better, one must look equally carefully at Vishnu-Krishna.

Thirdly, within yoga there is an extremely powerful tradition of the divinized guru, of a man become superman and in the process a living god on earth. Occasionally, as with Mahatma Gandhi, who saw himself as a karma-yogi, the guru is explicitly labelled an *avatar*. We therefore have to consider what it means to be a god descending into a mantle of flesh if we are also to consider what it means for a man to rise high enough to be called a god. Is it just possibly one and the same thing, in psychological terms?

An *avatara* is a 'descent', a down-coming or transference of a divine being into the world, a manifestation in the physical universe of a being whose essence and nature are not physical at all—a conception not unlike the incarnation of Christianity, the Word Made Flesh. The difference, however, is that whereas the Christian Logos appeared only once, avatar theory in Hinduism allows for multiple appearances. In fact, it is fundamental to Hinduism that the divine manifests itself often and variously in the flux of *maya*, and in the process there arise many objects, animals, fish, and birds as well as human beings which and who are special down-comings of divine substance. There is in effect a continuum of the divine-in-the material, from the idea that all is in some general sense God through various part-avatars—where one or other aspect of the divine is present in a sacred object, place, creature, or person—to the arch-avatars, as it were. These really-truly *avatars* signal a specific divine intervention in the affairs of the world or inaugurate a new age. In other words, the God who made the rules in the first place can calibrate his comings and goings in whatever way best pleases him.

The *avatar* concept is grandiose. As a model of how divinity behaves it is unique in the history of religions. It is a cumulative idea, in the sense that once one accepts that the cosmos might be run in such a way, one can go on adding to the vision all the time. The initial impetus to the theory arose when the two great Hindu epics, the *Mahabharata* and the *Ramayana*, were put into their current forms. These works were so huge and influential that a case was made for seeing them as a fifth *Veda*. This case was not successful—the *Vedas* remain only four in number—but few Hindus today read the *Vedas* while millions know the stories and the moral strictures of the epics. In these epics, two particular heroes stand out—Rama and Krishna—and both are widely conceived as *avatars* of Vishnu.

Once two such epic figures were accepted as descents of a great god, then in a universe of multiple rebirth, where divinity permeates the entire creation, it is easy to draw in a local god here, a famous hero there, a luminous saint elsewhere, and build up a firmament of *avatars*. Of the growth of the idea, Sampurnanand says:

The theory must have taken centuries to gain general acceptance. Even now it cannot be said to be an essential part of Hinduism. But it made several important additions to the Pantheon. Rama and Krishna, and to a lesser extent Nrisimha, are now objects of worship in their own right. Of course, it is admitted that they are incarnations or Avataras of Vishnu but a worshipper does not remind himself of this fact all the time. Taken all together, I am sure that there are more temples to Rama and Krishna than to Vishnu. Similarly, poetry, painting and sculpture have received more inspiration from Vishnu's Avataras than from him directly . . . Of course, any other god or goddess could manifest himself or herself as an Avatara, but Vishnu is the person with whose name the word has the strongest associations.[25]

Curiously enough, Krishna in the *Gita* does not say, 'Of course, I am Krishna here but Vishnu in my entirety.' He is a being called Krishna at every level, but tradition and inclination have made that particular entity a 'Vishnu' entity rather than, say, a 'Shiva' entity. In the mythology of the Hindus there is an enormous difference in personality and *style* between the two great gods or, if you will, the two ways of seeing God. Shiva's stories admit of no *avatars*: he is not born into flesh as anybody or anything, although he comes and goes in various forms. He is a far more fearsome being than Vishnu, although Vishnu is perfectly capable of being fierce and Shiva is perfectly capable of being tender. By his nature and by common consent, Vishnu is the kind of god who would incarnate from time to time in order to make life easier for mortals, where Shiva is not.

Generally, the *avatars* of Vishnu are conceived as players in a cosmic game, set pieces on a multi-dimensional chessboard who occur and recur in the cycle of the ages. Ten of them are singled out for special attention in the classical form of the theory, the *Dashavataras* who range from sub-human to superhuman as follows:

1. *Matsya avatara*   the fish avatar
2. *Kurma avatara*   the tortoise avatar
3. *Varaha avatara*   the boar avatar
4. *Narasimha avatara*   Nrisimha or Narsingh, the man-lion avatar
5. *Vamana avatara*   the dwarf avatar
6. *Parashurama avatara*   Parashurama, or Rama with the Axe
7. *Rama avatara*   Rama(chandra)
8. *Krishna avatara*   Krishna
9. EITHER
   Balarama avatara   Balarama
   OR
   Buddha avatara   Gautama the Buddha
10. *Kalki avatara*   Kalki(n), the avatar-to-come

In cosmic terms, these figures belong in the various *yugas* or world-ages: the first four are animal-centred avatars of the *Satya-yuga* or golden age, in symbolic terms not unlike the animal-headed deities of ancient Egypt; the next three are heroic males of the *Treta-yuga*, the third age, although Krishna is sometimes put in the second age or *Dvapara-yuga*. Buddha and Kalki belong in the fourth debased iron age, the *Kali-yuga*, in which we also live, after which the whole cycle is said to occur again. Certainly, there is an intriguing shift among the ten classical *avatars*. They move from remote cosmic animal symbols rather like signs of the Zodiac to more or less historical figures like Krishna and the Buddha, then back into fantasy with Kalki, the *avatar*-to-come, who will either be a horse or a brahmin riding a horse and carrying an apocalyptic sword.

The theory of *avatars* is not a static theory. It is open to reformulation, to claim and to counter-claim, and to extension in imaginative ways. In the middle of the Second World War, for example, certain Hindu pandits, aware of Nazi Aryan theories and the use of the swastika symbol, decided that Adolf Hitler was an avatar of Vishnu. He had come like Krishna at a time when the *dharma* was in danger—in this case specifically to bring about the downfall of the British Empire, an event that would deliver India from bondage. Which, indirectly, it did. A play in Hindi by Pandit Mahandas Dube was staged at Banaras Hindu University in 1942, entitled *Duskritavijaya* ('Victory over the Evil-doers'), in which Hita-lahare ('Wave of Benevolence'—Hitler) accompanied by Gaur-anga ('The Golden-Limbed'—Goering) burn Lankadahana (London) in the epic style of Rama attacking Lanka, the fortress of the demon-king Ravana.[26] For such virulently anti-British nationalists, the theme was perfectly reasonable; others such as Subhas Chandra Bose were already actually fighting on the Axis side against the occupying imperialists.

In 1966, Anakchandra Bhayawala, writing in a Bombay newspaper, argued that Charles Darwin was hardly the first to have proposed a theory of evolution. Rather, he was millennia late, because avatar theory *is* a theory of evolution. Bhayawala points out that the ten classic *avatars* are not so much descents by God as 'crossings-over' (another possible translation of *avatara*) from life in the water (fish) to animal life (boar) to half-human (man-lion) to primitive man (dwarf) to savage tool-maker (Rama with the axe) to moral man (Ramachandra) to civilized man (Krishna) to the truly superior philosopher (the Buddha) and, some day, to the super-being who will take our evolution further (Kalki).[27]

It is an elegant theory—or re-reading of the story.

Whatever form it takes, the theory of *avatars* demonstrates great vigour and attractiveness to all kinds of people. Mahatma Gandhi has been widely identified as an *avatar* of Vishnu, but not as far as I know equated with Kalki. Certainly, the symbolism of horse and sword hardly apply directly to the man whom Churchill called a 'half-naked fakir'.

When I lived in India I met Pitashree, who was according to his own claim and the belief of his followers the Brahmakumaris an *avatar* not of Vishnu but of Brahma. A few hundred yards from where he lived in his ashram on Mount Abu was the compound of another sectarian leader, who led the northern devotees of the early nineteenth-century saint Swaminarayan, who was conceived in his day as an *avatar* of Krishna. I met and spoke to the incumbent Swaminarayan, who proved to be a partial *avatar* in his own right of Krishna, who was the eighth classical *avatar* in *his* own right of Vishnu. The theory has a poetry all its own.

Hinduism is the most fluid of the great religions, so fluid that one often wonders whether it can be called a religion at all, or at least a single religion. A coolly clinical Western anthropologist might set about unpicking the skein, and eventually spread out all the strands neatly and say: 'That's it; that's what it really consists of.' A Western truth-seeker romanticizing the mystic East might exult in all the ambivalence, hype, dung, and divinity of modern India and declare that this is the ultimate reality and cosmic consciousness is on its way. Both will, however, meet their match, the anthropologist unable to resolve the panorama of fantasy into neat containers properly labelled, the devotee caught in an unexpected cold shower of logic and discipline. The relationship between human and deity is particularly susceptible to all the interplay of splendid nonsense and grubby truth one finds in India. Peter Brent, however, in *Godmen of India*, offers some clues as to what may be going on.

I mentioned the Swaminarayan sect a little earlier. Brent also encountered this movement, and wrote the following about its founder, who followed and adapted the doctrine of *vishishtadvaita* or qualified non-dualism proposed in the Middle Ages by Ramanuja:

An extra element in his thought, however, was the rather esoteric distinction he made between two aspects of Brahman, *akshara* and *purushottam*. The latter has been translated as 'highest of persons' and is considered supreme over mankind. The former, translated as an abstract 'imperishable', is seen as the abode, the physical body, of purushottam, which thus becomes the highest level of godhood. It is akshara (compared to which our cosmos is an ant to an elephant) with which the devotee must make contact in order to serve at the feet of purushottam itself. In coming to be known as Swaminarayan, Swami Sahajanand accepted that he was himself the incarnation of purushottam and is thus taken by his followers to have been a true avatar of God. This has given the sect a continuing intensity of devotion and supplied the spiritual power which has allowed generations of monks over nearly two centuries to live lives of such an extreme and restricted asceticism.[28]

The message here is clear, as indeed it is clear in other instances such as the case of Mahatma Gandhi. Adopting the mantle of avatarhood requires social interaction of some kind between the actual or potential avatar and a group of significant size. A little later, Brent quotes a follower of Swaminarayan on the nature of one's guru which adds another piece to the jigsaw:

The technique of the Guru is such, that even if he realizes that he has been flooded with all divinity, that God has just poured himself in him, the greater state beyond knowing this is that he has no consciousness of this knowledge. Supposing I know that I have been flooded by the ultimate divinity and that I represent God, then there is that 'I', and so 'I' is different from God. That subtle ego of being an emissary of God here comes in the way of one's own redemption as well as the redemption of all the disciples who come to me. But the state here is so subtle that the Guru who has been graced by God does not even have that consciousness.[29]

In other words, the relationship is conceived as non-egoistic, the guru being a vehicle of the divine without being or needing to be aware of it, or being aware of it in such a way as not to suffer from ego-bound arrogance. Anything else taints the potential relationship and one has, in effect, a failed avatar.

Many years ago in Scotland I met in the county of Argyll a woman called Sheena Govan who claimed to be the Second Christ and gained a brief newspaper-fed notoriety. She had several disciples, with one of whom I became friendly. Both Miss Govan and the disciple, Fred Astell, when not engaged upon their crusade, were by common agreement in the area intelligent, well-behaved, attractive people—nothing bizarre about them apart from the preposterous claim, around which the people who rather liked them as persons would circle with care. I liked them both and, despite the amusement of the press agency with which I was connected, found the most remarkable thing about them their patent sincerity. I was puzzled then and still remain fascinated by the *need* that some people have to feel touched by divinity, even singled out by it to special ends. Let me quote from my notes at the time:

'She is Christ, Tom,' Fred Astell said, after I had met her. 'I know as surely as you are sitting opposite me here. She is the same person, even in the flesh, though the features are smaller and feminine. I *know*. I've tried all the ologies and isms, gone up all the blind alleys, called myself a seeker after truth and a student of human nature and all the other fine names. But they are meaningless, because the truth is staring you in the face all the time.'

He had, he told me, known Christ before. In fact, the little group of disciples in the Highlands believed they were a coming together, a communal reincarnation, of Christ and his apostles as they once were in Palestine. He described how he first met her, in an open field on the island of Mull:

'We hadn't spoken a word, and yet I knew she was The Christ. She was surrounded by light, Tom. She stood there, with that light all around her, and as I watched I saw an image of Christ Himself merge with Her . . . How can I make you understand? I've seen her like that several times. It was beautiful, once, when she was walking away. And the majesty! No Shakespearian actor, no *human*, could have assumed such majesty as the being with whom she seemed blended.'

The group, however, did not thrive, the claim was dissipated, and Sheena Govan died some years later in relative peace and obscurity, never as far as I know invited to describe what had happened to her at that time—which is a pity. We are in the presence here of a phenomenon which is commoner than many might suppose: there are far more failed avatars, as it were, than those who have been 'recognized'. There is a psychology to avatarhood and avatar-recognition, which starts off in one-to-one relationships like *guru* and *shishya*, then must move to a collective stage if the whole adventure is to be ratified; that is, the proposition 'I am the incarnation of God' matched by the response 'Yes, I accept that you are the incarnation of God' has no value unless it moves to the stage where a large enough number of people are involved in belief and then act upon that belief in some way. 'By their fruits ye shall know them,' as the Bible has put it, or—more crudely—there must be evidence of earthly success. God must not only descend, but be known to have descended.

There is also an element of retroactive legislation in the establishment of avatars. Some individuals may state their claim confidently, others may hint at it with greater or less coyness or deviousness, others still may be acclaimed and then admit to it, and so forth. Additionally, however, someone in the past—mythic or historical—may be avatarized after the event and fitted into the system much as Mormons baptize their ancestors into Mormondom. This appears to be how the classical ten avatars were established, a system which does not in the least prevent all sorts of other assertions of avatarhood virtually all the time in India and often elsewhere as well where the word is not known but the phenomenon is just as common. In fact, we need the word to cover that universal phenomenon. The avatar and the messiah ought to become significant objects of sociological-anthropological study.

Whatever one believes about the divine and the human, there is overwhelming evidence that three easily blended phenomena regularly occur: someone claims godhead outright, godhead appears to claim someone, or godhead is claimed for someone during that person's lifetime or after death. The basic position may be complicated by using terms like 'prophethood' or 'messiahship' instead of 'godhead', but basically the phenomenon is the same. All such claims are more or less validated if and when they are accepted by enough people. How many claims, however, have fallen by the wayside, and how many people have found other means of coping with the syndrome that in some erupts as the avatar claim?

In a religion like Hinduism and, within it, in a system like yoga, everything is geared towards the regular appearance of humanized divinities and divinized humans, blending until the distinction between the two is lost and irrelevant. If generations of men (and sometimes women) have taken merger with the ultimate as their goal, with all sorts of special powers and prerequisites along the way, then inevitably some are going to succeed, or appear to succeed, or lay claim to having succeeded, or be said by others to have succeeded. Thus Swami X 'attained God-consciousness in such and such a year' and Sad-guru Y became identified with Brahman or Vishnu or Krishna after this or that profound experience. Yoga differs from more conventional religious-mystical-philosophical procedures in only one way but in that a most profound way: instead of waiting upon the grace of God in the fullness of time, yoga offers everyone on earth a do-it-yourself technology for becoming God.

It is small wonder then that the results are often bizarre and the paths followed often dangerous for mental stability; it is also small wonder that people are perennially fascinated by such a spiritual technology. The yogis have warned against the dangers, and have often themselves fallen into all the traps they have warned against. What remains, however, when all the detritus of delusion, deception and despair has been sifted through, is one of the most compelling facts of human history and culture: that such a self-transcending technology exists (however judged), and that it evolved within a society in which divine descents and human ascents are part and parcel of how things are. Hinduism in this is not at all like the Judaeo-Christian-Islamic tradition, built upon messiahs but admitting only one here or another there; in Hinduism the supply is so generous as to flood the system.

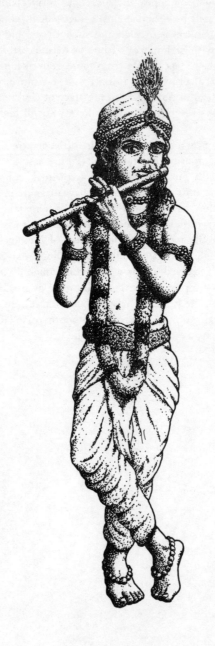

6. BHAKTI

Brindaban, India—The first shadows of dusk seem to bring this sacred old city to life with prayer. From its narrow, winding streets comes an eerie tinkling of cymbals, the buzz of chanting and the peal of bells.

The soft night air soon becomes fragrant with incense and sweets to be offered to Lord Krishna, one of the most popular gods of the Hindu pantheon. Thousands of years ago, Krishna's sensuous adolescent adventures are said to have taken place here on the banks of the Jumna River.

On the occasion of Krishna's birthday, on Sept. 7, tens of thousands of pilgrims flocked here. They were poor farmers, teachers, professionals and hundreds of mendicant holy men, or *sadhus*, with long matted hair, staffs and begging bowls.

'I became a sadhu to drink of God's sweet bliss,' said a bearded man in a tattered loincloth whose white hair was smeared with yellow dye as a symbol of his devotion. 'Here it is special because of Krishna. Here you can find peace.'

With these four short paragraphs Steven R. Weisman started a report on the 1985 *Krishnajayanti* celebrations in the city of Brindaban, between Delhi and Agra. Circulated by the *New York Times* news service, the report appeared in the *International Herald Tribune* on 16 September, a little over a week after these birthday celebrations for the eighth avatar of Vishnu. It was therefore a fresh commentary, an up-to-date description of a devotional enthusiasm that has if anything been increasing within Hinduism over the last two thousand years; certainly it has not diminished. As such, it is an eloquent testimony to both the continuity and the vitality of Hindu civilization, whether or not the West finds that civilization easy to understand.

Weisman's description includes all the scents, sounds, and sights of a Hindu festival; there are drums and cymbals, bells and harmoniums, the scent of flower-garlands, the chanting of mantras, the blowing of conch-shells, the distribution of sweet *prasad* to the devotees, the vivid calendar art, the processions, the dramatic enactments, the hands raised in *puja*, the flowers cast on altars, and the glowing myriad lamps at

night. All of it, together with the eager, exalted faces and the surging
crowds, makes up the reality of *bhakti*—the total surrender of self to
God.

Two closely linked words go back as far as there are records of the
Sanskrit language. The first of these is *bhaga* and the second is *bhakti*.
Both concern the idea of 'sharing'—of distribution, division, parts, and
wholes. Their spiritual overtones lead on to the idea of a divine Sharer-
Distributor, and to the homage paid to him by the receivers of those
shares. The two words also include the idea of good fortune, of one's lot
or portion in life, and of the love given by the husband or wife who is
also one's lot in life. They then become generalized love, and ultimately
the relationship between divine and human conceived as love, whether
that love is symbolized as between parent and child, between friends, or
between lovers.

There was, long ago, a Vedic god called Bhaga. He represented the
sharing out of property and the spoils of war once a year among the adult
men of the Indo-Aryan clans. Because he made no distinction between
these men he was conceived as blind—like Justice in the general
mythology of the West. In addition, he dispensed favours and presided
over love and marriage. This deity is at least one of the prototypes for
the later gods of the devotional cults that grew up around such divine
names as Bhagavat, Vasudeva, Narayana, Vishnu, Rama, and Krishna.
These cults were far less concerned with the ritual sacrifices of the
Vedic brahmins than with an immediate personal rapture; the raw and
potent emotions of the everyday—the kind that Gautama the Buddha
withdrew from—were in these movements to serve as they very means
of escaping birth and death. Song, dance, loud self-expression, visible
ecstasy, and crying the name of God would transform mortal desire into
something finer; the sweet bliss of human love, life, and sexuality would
be transmuted into 'God's sweet bliss', and the symbolic stories of
Krishna disporting with the *gopis* would serve to turn the devotee away
from earthly lusts towards the marvel of everlasting divine communion.

Nowadays in India *Bhagwan* is a common colloquial name for 'God'
or for a greatly revered human being whom God has touched. *Bhagwat*
may also refer to deity, but is more usually a name for the devotee,
derived from *bhagavat*, with its multitude of possible translations in
English: 'fortunate', 'blessed', 'adorable', 'venerable', 'divine',
'august', 'illustrious' and the like. In its compound form, it is the first
element in the phrase *Bhagavad-Gita*, which is often translated as 'The
Song of the Adorable One', or 'The Lord's Song', and could with equal
authenticity be 'The Divine Song' or 'The Song of the Blessed'. In
Sanskrit and the other Indian languages linked with it, that phrase has

far more cultural echoes than can ever by conveyed in English, and these echoes concern the meanings of *bhaga* and *bhakti*.

Bhakti probably originated in descriptions of the portions offered to the gods in a Vedic sacrifice, but by the time of the *Gita* it had become something else entirely—a *yoga* (technique of integration) or a *marga* (life-path). It should come as no surprise, after this etymological excursion, that a spiritual treatise called the *Bhagavad-Gita* could only serve, whatever nods it might make along the way to other yogas and life-paths, as a textbook of *bhakti*. The *Gita* describes and integrates into its complex whole a variety of philosophies and practices, but it has only one goal. Among these philosophies and practices it looks at, and admires, both *jnana-marga*, or the life-path of the Gnostic ('knowledge is the way') and *karma-marga*, the life-path of the Doer of Deeds ('action is what counts'). There is a place for them, but the highest life-path is *bhakti-marga*, the way of loyalty to and love for Krishna, by whatever name he is known. As K.M. Sen puts it:

Of the three Hindu religious paths, *jnana*, the path of knowledge, is apt to be dry and hard, and *karma*, the path of work (of religious performances), has often been exclusive. It is not surprising therefore that *bhakti*, the path of devotion, has enjoyed great popularity. The religious expression of this cult is in love and adoration, and it implies a belief in the Supreme Person rather than in a Supreme Abstraction. Naturally, this school of thought has not been much concerned with the intricacies of theology, and compared with the teachings of the *Upanishads*, the *Samkhya*, or the *Advaita Vedanta*, is less sophisticated. God is here looked upon as an intensely lovable Creator, and the *Bhakti* movement led to religious exuberance rather than to calm speculations about the all-pervading *Brahman*.[30]

By and large it is so, although one should not assume that behind popular *bhakti* there is no theology, or that the theologians of *bhakti* were any less willing to speculate and weave complexities than any other Hindu thinker. The *Gita* has a direct message, but it is an enormously complex work, as are such other *bhakti*-related treatises as the *Vishnu-Purana* and the *Bhagavata-Purana*. It is true to say, however, that the thinkers would accept the general unimportance of their systems when compared with *bhakti* self-surrender. It is the devotion itself that matters and leads to merger with the divine, not thinking about the devotion.

It is possible, as A.L. Basham maintains, that

the devotion (*bhakti*) of the early Bhagavatas, as exemplified in the *Bhagavad-Gita*, had been somewhat restrained in its expression. By the less spiritually developed worshipper the god was probably not thought of as an ever-present and indwelling spirit, but as a mighty and rather distant king, to be adored from afar . . . When Krsna reveals himself as the supreme god and shows his transcendent form, Arjuna falls to the ground in terror, unable to bear the awful splendour of the theophany. The god admittedly states that he is in the heart of all beings, that he raises his worshippers from the sea of transmigration, and that they are very dear to him; but he is still rather God Transcendent than God Immanent.[31]

The *Gita* was a propaganda document, designed to reconcile brahmin and kshatriya on the one hand and to help overcome the influence of Buddhism on the other; its aim was not to attack renunciation, the way of knowledge or the way of selfless service, but to transcend it. As a consequence it is a work whose exuberance is tempered with the moderation it recommends, so that it may seem less vivid and vehement than many later *bhakti* tracts. It should be borne in mind, however, that *Krishnabhaktas* (the devotees of Krishna) have never thought of it as a bit of religious diplomacy, an anti-Buddhist text, or even an exemplar of moderation, and there is enough vitality in it to satisfy them fully. In sum, they take it as their principal text and justification, in which Krishna reveals himself and talks directly to us all. For them, Krishna the charioteer of the *Gita* is Krishna the flute-player in the Garden of Brindaban, the Krishna venerated by Chaitanya in sixteenth-century Bengal, and honoured in the chants of the Krishna-consciousness Movement throughout the world today. And *that* Krishna is both transcendent *and* immanent, a warm sea of love in whom to submerge oneself.*

Today the *Gita* is the most popular religious-mystical work among the Hindus and the best-known of all the Hindu classics to the world at large. It is embedded like a jewel in the larger mass of the epic *Mahabharata*, much as the Gospels are embedded in the Bible; it has 18 chapters and 700 verses in its own right, but is only an episode—Book VI—in the vast landscape of the epic. The date of the work is uncertain. Some authorities allow themselves plenty of latitude, arguing that it is not earlier than the rise of Buddhism (*c*.500 BC) and not later than the rise of the great devotional cults (*c*.500 AD), when the tide had begun to turn against Buddhism in India. With Sen, however, I am inclined to believe that the composition took place between 400 and 200 BC, as a direct response to the success of the Buddhists, but some authorities consider it of an age with the Gospels, while many orthodox Hindus insist that it is *at least* 3,000 years old.

*There is a fuller review of the *Gita*, together with an easy-to-read prose version, in my *Yoga and the Bhagavad-Gita* (Aquarian Press, 1986).

Paradoxes abound in this primary textbook of both *yoga* and the *bhakti-marga*. It preaches love and moderation in the brief prelude to a bloody battle, and the god of love urges Prince Arjuna to do his share of slaughter in that battle. Mohandas Karamchand Gandhi took it to be a work of pacifism and a bible of passive resistance to the British; his assassin Nathuram Godse found in it the conviction necessary in order to kill *him*. The story is highly artificial and stylized, yet at the same time haunting and full of charm, so much so that one cannot say how many translations have been made into the languages of the West, although in English alone there are more than fifty.

Bhakti is a democratic or populist movement. The brahmin philosophers, like Ramanuja in the Middle Ages, who helped to disseminate it and make it theologically respectable, were inclined to sustain the distinctions of caste, and yet the *Gita* and other works emphasize the universality of the message and the accessibility of both the path and the God to whom the path would lead. It is as open to women as to men, to children as to adults, to low caste as to high, to poor as to rich, and it does not usually make enormous ascetic or intellectual demands. It requires no *asanas* or other bodily practices, but does demand the chanting of *mantras*, meditation upon *murtis* (images), and great personal dedication to the Lord, whatever his favoured name. This dedication can take many forms, summed up in the following, from Peter Brent's *Godmen of India*:

Although in a religion as eclectic as Hinduism divisions tend to blur and labels to become meaningless, two main streams may be said to run through it. The first is the Shaivite, devoted to Shiva, the tenor of which is ascetic and self-mortifying. Those sadhus who distort and sometimes cripple their bodies with austerities of the most extreme kind are nearly always Shaivites. The second stream, that of the Vaishnavites, lays no such stress on self-torture. Worshipping Vishnu in his incarnation as Krishna, they prefer that happy god's lightness of heart, his emphasis on the pleasures of the senses as a metaphor for the pleasures of the spirit. They are bhaktas, followers of the way of love and devotion and tend to be anti-Brahminical, to disbelieve in the total merging of the individual soul with Brahman, to use vernacular languages rather than Sanskrit, to focus their faith through idols, to delight in ritual . . .

The gopis of Vrindaban, the dairymaids who tended the cows and sported—in pure or in ambivalent manner, according to the tale you choose—with the young Krishna, are the clearest example of those who follow the pushti-marg [the pathway of the love of God]. They joined in the lila of God, in his game, his sport, and to do so remains the highest aim of the devotees of Krishna. He is the husband of all souls and every soul aspires to join with him in divine bliss. As a result, the enactment of the love games between Krishna and the cow girls becomes a holy rite of great significance . . . [He then quotes:]

'Vallabhacharya's [a sixteenth-century guru] God is the child of your home; you can worship him as a child. The adoration which we have for a child . . . if we can give that same love to Lord Krishna, or if we worship Lord Krishna as our friend, then that's all right, he has got so many friends. There are even so many fellows worshipping him as their beloved. We have got so much love for God—for his love, you see—we can discard our husbands or our elders so that love can be given to God.'[32]

Love and sexual symbolism permeate the bhakti cults in a variety of ways. A story is told, for example, of the sage Narada who became tired of celibacy and went to Krishna with a request.

'You have 16,008 wives,' he said. 'That is too many even for a god. I am tired of being a bachelor. Could you not perhaps in your kindness spare me just one of your wives?'

'By all means,' said Krishna. 'Go to my ladies' apartments, and take for yourself the first one you find who is not occupied with me.'

Puzzled but pleased, Narada went to the ladies' apartments, and entered the room of Krishna's principal wife—but there he found Krishna enjoying her company. He was surprised, having just left his divine friend, but he was not too perturbed. There were plenty more. He then went to the next room, but here too he saw Krishna, enjoying his second wife. Narada, it is said, went to every room but came away baffled and still a bachelor, because Krishna was with each wife in every one of the 16,008 rooms.

And that is the essence of *bhakti*. The Lord has many friends, and love enough for all of them.

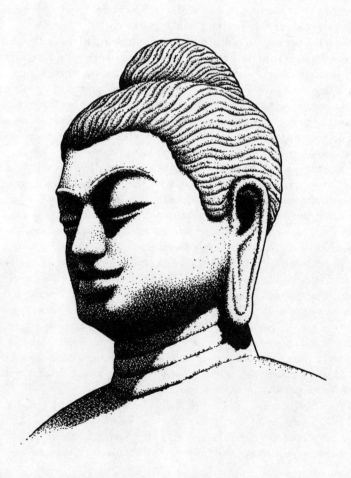

7. BUDDHI and BUDDHA

Sagara, king of Ayodhya, had lost a horse. It was no ordinary horse, but part of a great sacrifice by means of which he hoped to wrest dominion of the world from Indra, king of the gods.

Indra, however, had spirited the horse away beneath the earth, where it wandered near to the hermitage of the sage called Kapila. King Sagara set his thousands of sons digging in order to find the horse again, and they dug with such vigour that the earth herself protested against the violation. Indra, however, told her to be calm, assuring her that soon the brood of princelings would meet their match. In the meantime, on and down they dug, until they broke through into that remote place where the horse grazed and Kapila sat wrapt in meditation.

The many sons of Sagara were not a quiet lot. They rushed towards the horse, refused to do obeisance to the sage, and even began to believe that he had stolen the animal in the first place. Some stormed towards him too, shouting and raising their weapons. As they did so, however, the meditating sage opened his eyes—and reduced every member of the royal multitude to ashes.

Kapila means 'the reddish one', both the colour of certain monkeys and of fire and the sun. The story, marvellously fantastic in the spirit of Hindu myth, symbolizes how the blaze of ultimate reality can reduce the riot of *maya* to nothingness, and fits in perfectly with other tales of gods and yogis demolishing troublemakers with a single fiery glance. There was, however, a flesh-and-blood historical Kapila, who lived when the forest sages of ancient India were reshaping the message of the *Vedas* and blending into it the philosophy of the warrior caste and of the pre-Aryan peoples of the subcontinent.

Although his name is not at all well known in the West, Kapila is one of the founders of the philosophy on which yoga is based. His description of the cosmos—known as the *Sankhya* ('Numbers')—has been universally recognized for some two thousand years in India as the sister discipline to Patanjali's Yoga: the theoretical wing of a subject for which Patanjali provided the practical wing. *Sankhya* is a complex and subtle system that pervades much of Hindu thought and can be found liberally scattered through, and recognized in, the *Bhagavad-Gita*. Along with Patanjali's Yoga, it is one of the *Shaddarshanas* or six classical systems of philosophy within orthodox Hinduism, to be contrasted with Jainism and Buddhism, the two main heterodox systems. This conflict and contrast between the orthodox or *astika* and the heterodox or *nastika* is significant in view of what follows.

Little is known about the historical Kapila. According to tradition, his father Kardama was also a *rishi* or sage but, importantly, it was from his mother Devahuti that he learned the fundamentals of his philosophy and ideas about matter and spirit. He appears to have lived where modern Nepal meets the Indian state of Bihar; in this region his disciples built a city in his honour, Kapilavastu, but in later life he went to an island in the mouth of the Ganges, not far from present-day Calcutta, where he meditated and taught. Its name is Sagara, the same as the king of Ayodhya whose sons he incinerated at a glance; the word means 'sea' or 'lake', and every year to this day, in late January, early February, devotees still go there to honour his memory. He is listed in the *Bhagavata Purana* as one of the 21 avatars of the god Vishnu.

Of the times in which Kapila lived, the cultural anthropologist Joseph Campbell has written:

We may register, then, with a glance again at Greece beyond the other bound of the Persian Empire, a gradual rise and flowering from c. 800 to c. 500 B.C. of a multitude of . . . monarchic states across the whole domain from Athens to Bengal: literally hundreds of tiny sovereign powers, each with its capital fortress, town, or city, governed by a princely family and with councils of elders, citizen assemblies, palace army, temple clergy, peasantry and trading gentry, shops, dwellings and—among the more prosperous— monuments and parks. And behold, at a certain time there began appearing in these pleasant little capitals wandering teaching sages, each with his cluster of devotees and each supposing himself to have solved—once and for all—the mystery of sorrow: Kapila (perhaps c. 600 B.C.), Gosala (fl. 535 B.C.), Mahavira (d. 485 B.C.), the Buddha (563–483 B.C.), Pythagoras (c. 582–500 B.C.), Xenophanes and Parmenides (both, also, of the sixth century), and Empedocles (c. 500–430 B.C.)[33]

Many scholars and historians have commented rather wonderingly on the rise of the philosopher-mystics of that period, and along with them many of the root ideas of the modern world. Some have even gone so far as to suggest (Julian Jaynes, for example) that around this time a new kind of mentality or consciousness may have become available to the human race, Jaynes being particularly attracted to the idea of a new integration between the hemispheres of the brain.[34] However that may be, the sages themselves—in esoteric teachings for the few or popular systems for the masses—believed that they were offering a new awareness that transcended old ritualism and sacred hierarchies. Foremost among them, Kapila not only founded his Sankhya on rationality, but promoted a three-part model of the human mind that is still the accepted Hindu theory today.

Uppermost in his tripartite *chitta* or 'mindstuff' was the quality called *buddhi*, present in the universe as Mahat or 'the Great One' and as 'awakeness' in each individual. *Buddhi* illuminates everything below it in human nature, and is closest to the *jiva* or living spirit (*atman* in the *Upanishads*) that witnesses everything and, in its subtle sheath, passes from life to life and death to death. Below *buddhi* comes *ahamkara*, the ego-former, the quality of mind that says 'I am me' and sustains the idea of separateness and individuation. Below *ahamkara* is *manas*, the mechanical mind that like a charioteer uses the reins of the senses to drive the body-chariot through the world.

The Sankhya-Yoga concept of a three-layered mind is fascinating in its own right, but doubly fascinating because, in the twentieth century, Western theorists have begun to propose three-layer minds and brains. Sigmund Freud's model is well known now, with the Super-ego above, the Ego in the middle, and the Id underneath. It is a psychoanalytic picture offered to help account for kinds of behaviour, whether conscious or unconscious; it does not have anything to say about intelligence or the autonomic nervous system, but it is a model of the mind none the less. Less well known but equally interesting is the Papez-Maclean biological model, which proposes three layers of the physical brain that conform to three distinct stages in the evolution of the human being. Lowest is the reptilian brain, a primitive centre for all sorts of basic drives and processes; above it the mammalian mid-brain builds a more complex and sophisticated structure of drives and processes onto its base, and then is capped by the forebrain or neocortex with its great hemispheric divisions. This third level is the seat of truly human intelligence.[35]

We do not know much about the brain, and know even less about the mind; what investigators have begun to learn is promising, but it is all still at a stage not far removed from the models of ancient thinkers like Kapila. The similarity among all three models just described, however, must make us both uneasy and reverent: there is a great deal of confusion in and around subjects like yoga, but time and again one comes back to incontestable gems like these.

Kapila's theory is powerful because it asserts that each 'individual' human being is in fact a 'multiple' human being. This appears to be a universal conclusion about personality among mystics of many backgrounds, and the strongest argument in favour of systems like yoga which seek to transcend the warring multiplicity in each of us and 'unite', 'unify', or 'integrate' our personalities. However we were created—in the slow trial and error of evolution or by a god scooping up clay—we appear to be in real need of integrative techniques, whether to get off a miserable wheel of birth and death or to help biological-cum-social evolution on its way to better things.

Kapila was typical of his time, however, in that he taught the essentially miserable nature of existence. This misery arises out of three conditions: the intrinsic disorder of mind and body; extrinsic misfortunes coming at each of us from the world Out There, in the form of people, animals, or natural disaster; and thirdly, the impact of the supernatural, the wilfulness of gods, demons, atmosphere, and heavenly bodies. The Sankhya system arose to describe how this universal state of affairs was to be rationally interpreted, while the Yoga system of Patanjali arose to offer an austere but manageable personal technology for overcoming the problems. Both no doubt took centuries to reach the forms in which they have come down to us, but while they were doing so another thinker appeared in the same tradition as Kapila to take the problems and the solutions further, and to weave his own doctrine of what it is to be truly 'awake'.

'What are you then?' a brahmin once said to the kshatriya called Siddhartha Gautama, prince of the Shakya clan. 'Are you a god, a demigod, a spirit, or a man?'

'None of these,' said Gautama. 'I am a buddha.'

An awakened one—a special category of being into whom the light of reality shines unimpeded. There have been arguments about whether Gautama the Buddha ever existed, just as there have been arguments about the historicity of Jesus Christ. Certainly the fantasy thinking of myth and parable surrounds them both; but all the evidence points to real men in real time, each of whom changed the world inordinately just by being there.

Siddhartha Gautama was born in the land of Magadha, where modern Nepal and the Indian state of Bihar meet. He was the son of Suddhodana, governor or *raja* of a province in the kingdom of Kosala, and Suddhodana's capital was the city of Kapilavastu, perhaps only a century after it was built, and certainly at a time when Kapila's fame and teachings were still seminal there. Gautama's life, especially his early life, is festooned with myth, but the myth is as important as any

historical detail we may have about how he and his buddhahood
developed. Legend says, for example, that the boy was marked from
birth as either a world emperor or a world teacher. His father
Suddhodana preferred the former, and is supposed to have tried to
shield his son from every influence that might send his thoughts in the
direction of mysticism and austerity. Young Siddhartha was competent
in arms but not enthusiastic about war; he accepted and enjoyed his wife
Yashodhara, and benefited from the pleasures of palace and park, where
the ills of the world did not reach. Until, as the story goes, the Four
Signs occurred.

When Gautama made it clear that he wanted to see more of the real
world, his father had the roads and the city cleaned and decorated in
order to keep the unsightly at bay. With his faithful charioteer Channa,
Prince Gautama went forth, and in spite of all his father's precautions
saw on the first day an old feeble man with swollen veins, broken teeth,
wrinkled skin, and trembling limbs.

'What kind of being is that?' he asked.

'They call it an old man,' said Channa.

'What is *old*?' asked the prince.

'Old,' said the charioteer, 'is the loss of life. It is decay of mind and
memory. It is the slow approach of death.'

On the second day Prince Gautama went forth, and this time he saw a
sick man—feverish, exhausted, and smeared with his own dung—
breathing with difficulty and without either friends or shelter.

'What kind of being is that?' he asked.

'They call it a sick man,' said Channa.

'What is *sick*?' asked the prince.

'Sick,' said the charioteer, 'is loss of health. It too can lead to death.'

On the third day Prince Gautama went forth, and this time he saw a
dead body being carried on a bier as if on a bed, dressed in strange
garments and accompanied by weeping people.

'Who or what is this?' he asked.

'It is a dead man,' said Channa. 'He has no further need of anything or
anyone here. Like a ruined wall or a fallen leaf he is cut off forever from
father and mother, brother and sister, child and kin. Siddhartha, you
too will die.'

On the fourth day, when prince Gautama went out, he saw a holy
man in a robe of yellow cloth standing by the wayside. The man looked
calmly at him, and held out a begging bowl.

'Who is this?' he asked.

'He is a holy man,' said the charioteer. 'He restrains his appetites and
his desires, does no harm to anyone and is full of sympathy for all
creatures.'

The prince felt a great longing to be like that holy man, but when he returned that day to the palace the birth of his son was announced, and immediately he became involved again in the life of a householder. He had, however, learned revulsion for the imperfections of this world, and had seen a possible way of release. Dutifully he told his father about his experiences and his thoughts, and in sudden dread Suddhodana doubled the guards and urged the dancing girls of the palace to redouble their revels.

It was all to no avail, of course: neither sense of caste duty, nor wife, nor son, nor dancing girls held Gautama back when the time came to leave. One night he fled away, accompanied only by Channa as far as the river Anoma. Channa in tears begged him to return or—if he was resolved—to let him go with him, but the prince refused.

'Not yet,' he said. 'You must go back and tell my father not to grieve for me.'

He then crossed the river to his new life, and wandered for seven years until in frustration he chose to wander no further. He had sat at the feet of learned brahmins and found them not learned enough; he had performed severe austerities with Jain recluses, and found them too austere. But like the saints of the Jains who starved themselves to death rather than continue in the squalor of this world's activities, he came at last to a noble fig-tree (known still as the *ficus religiosa*), and resolved to sit there until either he knew the secret of suffering and release, or died in the attempt. This was at the place now called Sarnath, and the tree the Bodhi tree that has given its name to Bodhgaya.

Bodhi derives from the same root as *buddhi* and *buddha*. It is the enlightenment that people talk about when they call the Buddha 'The Enlightened One'. It was what the Buddha himself meant when he answered the brahmin. Someone possessed of *bodhi* was different.

But how different? Traditions both Hindu and Buddhist indicate that someone who has 'attained' is not simply and suddenly transformed; they uniformly insist that what people like Gautama achieved in the one life we know about had been climbing steadily through innumerable earlier lives to get there; indeed, there is a whole sub-tradition of Buddhism that tells fantasy tales about the Buddha-to-be (or *bodhisattva*) in his previous and preparatory lives. In crude general terms, nobody gets the last great lift into buddhahood as if it were a one-life-and-one-only kind of shortcut. Yoga, many will aver, can shorten the whole painful chore, but not *that* much, and here we come up against the rock-hard Indian conviction that the world is indeed a long, slow, painful experience—even for the Buddhas who teach a middle way between brahmin ritual and worldliness on one side and Jain negativism and self-torture on the other.

Let us leave aside for a moment, however, the issue of reincarnation and the awful wheel of birth and death. It is clear from Hindu and Buddhist texts that Hindus and Buddhists worry about death and dissolution just as much as human beings in any other system or part of the world. The larger vista of many lives is more impressive perhaps, but it is no more oppressive than, say, the traditional Christian horror of an eternity in hell or limbo. The epic pictures of death and of existence after death in both cultures are equally lurid and disquieting, while in both cultures the pain of existence is equally distressing. Thus, it is safe to conclude that, quite apart from who offers the better picture of reality or whether the idea of 'better pictures' is absurd, the main aim of all mystics everywhere is simply to cope more successfully with what happens to them in *this* world. They want to cope better than others around them cope, and they want to reach a point where coping is no longer an issue.

In essence, that is what yoga and all the other pragmatic religious-cum-mystical systems are *for*. And in the development of techniques for coping among sages like Kapila and Gautama, the concepts of *buddhi*, *buddha*, and *bodhi* are crucial, because they argue that the essence of coping better is being more awake, seeing more light without being blinded. Whether in their myths or in their logical systems, the solution always finally rests where *buddhi* is conceived to be: in the top of the head, at the top of the layers of the mind, in the skull where the third eye can be found, or in the thousand-petalled lotus that opens when the kundalini rises from the mud of the genitals to the heaven of realization.

In the head.

Patanjali states the situation clearly enough: the purpose of yoga is *chittavritti-nirodhah*—'stilling the ripples of the mind', all of the mindstuff down below being enlightened by what pours in through *buddhi*. The *atman*, the 'spirit' that lies beyond, is not active in this; it never changes, is involved yet not involved. *Buddhi* is the crucial element in the sheer intellectuality of Sankhya and Yoga, of both the Eight-fold path (*ashthangika-marga*) of the Buddha and its cousin the Eight-limb yoga (*ashthanga-yoga*) of Patanjali. The *Gita* is not entirely convinced about them, however, because it introduces a higher factor (in the view of its compilers). That factor is *bhakti*, personal devotion and surrender to a personal God. Neither Kapila nor Patanjali nor Gautama takes a personal God as central or even relevant in their rational schemes; over one life or over many, you get there by following an intellectual regime that opens up the head to enlightenment. In the *Gita* that is recognized as possible—just—but greater success is to be achieved there by opening up the heart.

These are the extremes within the ancient systems that underlie later yoga or yogas: the tug-of-war between *buddhi* in the head and *bhakti* in the heart.

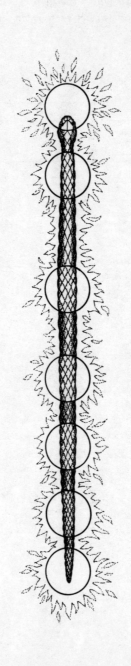

8. CHAKRA and KUNDALINI

'I asked a great Mahatma,' wrote Shree Purohit Swami in 1938, 'what would awaken the kundalinee and he said; "Renunciation, Renunciation, Renunciation", and I found it true. I met some Hatha-Yogis who through postures and breathing exercises awakened the kundalinee, but as soon as they left their meditative life, the passage closed again. It is the inner fire, the serpentine fire, as it is called, that leads a man to liberation, that makes the mind fit for concentration, and the body fit to sustain the weight of the higher spiritual powers.

'It is a terrifying experience when the kundalinee is awakened. The first day the fire was kindled in me, I thought I was dying, the whole body was, as it were, on fire, mind was being broken to pieces, the bones were being hammered, I did not understand what was happening. In three months I drank gallons of milk and clarified butter, ate leaves of two nimba trees till they were left without a single leaf, searched everywhere for the mudra leaves and devoured those insipid things. During that period I could not sit in any posture, I could not stand, I used to lie down on my bed and repeat the name of Lord Dattatreya. I know of cases where the fire was not brought under control for six or eight months; one mahatma told me that he used to sit under a cold water tap for eight hours every day. There is no danger to life, unless the rules and discipline are disregarded; it is only an act of purification, through which everyone must go if he wants to attain.'[36]

'There was a sound like a nerve thread snapping,' wrote Gopi Krishna in 1971, 'and instantaneously a silvery streak passed zigzag through the spinal cord, exactly like the sinuous movement of a white serpent in rapid flight, pouring an effulgent, cascading shower of brilliant vital energy into my brain, filling my head with a blissful lustre in place of the flame that had been tormenting me for the last three hours. Completely taken by surprise at this sudden transformation of the fiery current, darting across the entire network of my nerves only a moment before, and overjoyed at the cessation of pain, I remained absolutely quiet and motionless for some time, tasting the bliss of relief with a mind flooded with emotion, unable to believe I was really free of the horror.'[37]

The serpent power called *kundalini-shakti*, along with the centres through which it is said to ascend from the anus to the crown of the head, is one of the most remarkable and confusing features of yoga. There are many reasons for this, but sufficient to start off with is a simple contrast between the two vivid and dramatic descriptions just given and the following from Swami Gnaneswarananda of the Ramakrishna Mission:

As soon as the *kundalini* is stirred up, something like a combustion takes place which generates, in a very subtle spiritual sense, heat and light at the base of the *sushumna*. With the awakening of the *kundalini* the yogi actually feels a unique and soothing heat and light at the base of his spine. The awakened kundalini is then made to travel upwards by means of a highly symbolic form of meditation which unfolds higher and higher spiritual qualities in man.[38]

Heat is present in all three descriptions, but whereas the first two are wild, agonizing and ultimately ecstatic accounts, the third is calm and much more in line with the disciplined qualities one expects from yoga. At the same time, however, all three agree upon an alternative anatomy and physiology of the body to what Western science and medicine accept, in which not just heat but *light* of some kind can develop in the buttocks.

To begin any kind of discussion of this most alien aspect of yoga one needs to place it in historical and regional context. It arises out of Tantrism, whose classic centre in the early Middle Ages was Bengal. Tantra is one of the truly ancient traditions of India, shared by both Hinduism and Buddhism, but bearing little direct relationship either with the Vedic orthodoxy of Hinduism or the standard teachings of Buddhism. It has tended to be exotic, occult, and mysterious—indeed, it is not considered entirely respectable even today in India, although Tantric ideas suffuse the whole of popular and philosophical Hinduism.

Secondly, inside Tantrism, the two schools of *laya-yoga* ('the way of dissolution') and *hatha-yoga* ('the way of force') have had close ties, and it is in laya-yoga that the theory and practice of a goddess-like power moving through the channels of the body has reached its fullest development. Today, because of the cross-fertilization of yoga with yoga, the idea of serpent powers and subtle centres is mixed in with many other traditions, but it is worth stressing that the concept of a special anatomy and physiology is virtually non-existent in the classical Upanishads, in Kapila's Sankhya, in Patanjali, and in the *Gita*. The

Katha-Upanishad mentions body currents, one of which rises to the head, and the *Gita* talks of centring the prana between the brows, but that is about all. In his *Raja Yoga*, Vivekananda interweaves the idea of *kundalini* with his commentary on the *Yoga-sutras*. For him, a Bengali whose movement, the Ramakrishna Mission, has strong Tantric roots, this was a natural tie-in, but for many orthodox Hindus the tie-in does not appear to have been natural, or even possible.

As will become clear, this is fiercely controversial territory, particularly because, as Georg Feuerstein points out, the experience of the risen serpent 'is supposed to differ essentially from its equivalent in non-tantric schools . . . The rousing of the latent force within the body and its controlled guidance upwards through the six centres is claimed to lead to a more complete enlightenment than is the case with ordinary Yoga.'[39] In other words, all enlightenments are equal, but one is more equal than the others—*and* that one is more focused on the body than the others.

In Sanskrit, *kunda* is a jar or a pot, or a fire pit in the ground. A *kundala* is a ring, a coil, or a snake, and so the feminine derivative *kundalini* is both a fiery container and a coiled-up serpent. It is also a *devi* or goddess, the equivalent inside the body of the vast and powerful goddess Shakti who pervades the created universe— who *is* the created universe. Separately, a *chakra* is something that runs and turns, the wheel of a chariot or for making pots. In symbolic terms it is also a mystical circular diagram and a circle of dominion, so that a *chakravarti(n)* is a world emperor. And lastly, a *padma* is a lotus, the Indian waterlily that symbolizes spiritual purity and aspiration, rising on its slender stem from the mud of the world, its roots under the water of life.

The Tantric picture of our inner anatomy and physiology is complex, but essentially it is said that in each of us the latent female snake lies coiled at the base of the spine around the lowest of the *chakras* or *padmas*. Between this lowest *chakra* and the highest there stretch entwined along the spine three subtle *nadis* (translated variously as 'nerves', 'veins', 'currents', or 'channels'). Two, the *ida* and the *pingala*, channel a kind of alternating current up and down the spine, associated with the inhalation and exhalation of the breath of life called *prana*. The third, however, is straight and sheath-like, with further subtler threads inside it, and goes direct from anus to crown. It is the *sushumna-nadi*, and in the normal way of things it is blocked off by the detritus of spiritual inefficiency.

The breathing and meditative practices of hatha- and laya-yoga can, however, purify and open this innermost spinal channel, and at the same time awaken the sleeping goddess. The practitioner should, most

preferably, be celibate, because in effect what happens is that natural
sexual energy is converted into a kind of psychic force and (though
conceived as feminine) rises with phallic strength upwards through the
sushumna. It may reach only to one or other of the intermediate *chakras*,
each with its quota of spiritual power, or it may go in a vigorous rush
right to the seventh *chakra* at or just beyond the crown of the head,
where a mystical union takes place between the goddess Kundalini-
Shakti and the god Shiva. *That* is the liberation beyond other liberations.
Of it, A.L. Basham says:

The awakened kundalini gives the yogi superhuman power and knowledge, and
many yogis have practised yoga rather for this than for salvation. Some adepts
of yoga have developed certain powers which cannot fully be accounted for by
European medical science, and which cannot be explained away as subjective,
but the physiological basis of laya- and hatha-yoga is certainly false: there is no
kuṇḍalini, suṣumṇa or *sahasrāra*. The ancient mystical physiology of India needs
further study, not only by professional Indologists, but by open-minded
biologists and psychologists, who may reveal the true secret of the yogi.[40]

That is the voice of friendly but sceptical Western scholarship. Other
Westerners are by no means as sceptical, as for example Peter Rendel
when he says:

One must learn to recognize these different principles or levels within oneself;
in other words learn to distinguish the finer from the grosser. Therefore one
must learn to work with and control the energies in oneself. Eventually one
comes to realize that all Life, including oneself, is just energy in different states
or in different states of vibration. These energies in one's own system are what
the chakras are all about. The chakras are the vital force centres at the different
levels of experience or consciousness in the human system . . . At a later stage
the highly evolved soul learns to control the powerful awakened energies which
flow through his system. He will be able to direct them upwards or downwards,
or focus them at whatever level he requires. For some people the effect of the
sublimation of the awakened kundalini will be one of rejuvenation. One is
reminded of Rider Haggard's 'She' who preserved the prime of her body by
bathing in the sacred fire in the mountain. It is interesting to speculate how
much the author knew of the esoteric aspect of his subject concerning the real
sacred fire within.[41]

Where Basham is the interested but objective Western scholar,
Rendel is the convinced Western occultist—the gnostic who knows a
higher truth, and ties Tantra in with 'the Western Mystery tradition',
with astrology, with Isis and Osiris, the Jewish Qabalah, and with
theosophy. Such occultists regularly draw parallels between Eastern and
Western mystical traditions, often to the point of suggesting that they
are one and the same tradition, and all part of a Great Design.

Anyone who wishes to gain a clear picture of the whole subject must therefore come to terms with four distinct centres of influence at work on books and articles written about the *chakras*, and in any course that may offer to awaken the sleeping serpent. Diagrammatically these are:

Assertions made by some Hindus about the truth and value of *laya-yoga*, etc.

Enthusiastic adoption of the theory and the practice of *laya-yoga* by Western occultists who are also interested in Eastern mysticism.

Doubts expressed by other Hindus about the wisdom of becoming involved in such practices, together with their absence from certain major works on yoga.

Cautious interest expressed by sceptical but open-minded scholars and scientists trained in Western methods (not to mention bafflement, amusement or outrage on the part of their colleagues who think the whole thing absurd).

These appear to be the inescapable ground rules of any discussion about the subtle energy centres. What, however, are the *chakras* themselves in detail?

Leaving aside certain inconsistencies as regards their number, nature, location, and relative importance, the general consensus appears to be that there are six way-station *chakras* linked with the spine and on the way to a seventh supreme *chakra*. In order, from the lowest to the highest, these seven are:

1. The *muladhara-chakra* or 'root-support-wheel'

Located in the area of the perineum, in the pelvic region just above the anus, this centre is linked with the element earth and is conceived as a yellow lotus with four red petals. In the heart of the lotus is the symbolic *yoni* or vagina, where the coiled energy lies. Its sense is smell, its mantra LAM, and its resident deity Dakini the Witch. Its function is cohesiveness and accumulation.

2. The *svadishtana-chakra* or 'self-standing-wheel'

Located a little above, in the area of the genitals, this centre is linked with the element water and is conceived as a white lotus with six red petals and a crescent in its core. Its sense is taste, its mantra VAM, and its resident deity Rakini. Its function is contraction.

3. The *manipura-chakra* or 'wheel of the city of jewels'

Located at the navel, this centre is linked with the element fire and is conceived as a scarlet lotus with ten golden petals. Its sense is sight, its mantra RAM, and its resident deity the virtuous goddess Lakini. Its function is expansion.

4. The *anahata-chakra* or 'wheel of the unstruck sound'

Located near the heart and often spoken of in English as the 'heart centre', it is linked with the element air and is conceived as a smoky or blue lotus with twelve flaming red petals. The breath of life dwells there and it gives forth the mystical unstruck inner sound. Its sense is touch, its mantra YAM, and its resident diety is Kakini the She-crow. Its function is movement, and it fosters the ego-sense.

5. The *vishuddhi-chakra* or 'wheel of great purity'

Located in the throat, this centre is linked with the element *akasha* ('ether' or space, the fifth Hindu element) and is conceived as a white or smoky lotus with sixteen petals. Its sense is hearing, its mantra HAM, and its resident deity is Shakini the Leafed One. Its function is to be spacious.

6. The *ajna-chakra* or 'wheel of insight'

Located between the eyebrows, it is the third eye of Shiva. It lies beyond the elements and is conceived as a lotus with no colour at all and only two petals. No senses attach to it, its mantra is AUM, and its resident diety Hakini. It is the *bindu* or point between the manifest and the unmanifest; it is *Mahat* and *buddhi*, supreme intellect, the point where consciousness begins to awaken and expand.

7. The *sahasrara-chakra* or 'wheel of a thousand'

Located either in the brain or just beyond the crown of the head, it is the goal of the risen *kundalini* and is conceived as a lotus with a thousand petals set in an ocean of light. It is union and liberation, the marriage of Shakti with Shiva and represents transcendental reality.

This list is more complex than many provided in Western books, but is still less complex than it might have been. One could, for example, add in the devanagari symbols inscribed on the petals of the lotuses, and the sages and spiritual tokens associated with each *chakra*, and the advantages said to be gained by meditating upon each of the centres. That, however, would have complicated an already complex matter. There is much in yoga and Hinduism that is alien and hard for Western minds to cope with, but there cannot be much that is more mystifying than the chakric ensemble. It enchants some, repels others, and causes many more just to shake their heads. And the more one attempts an explanation, the more the heads shake.

There is some consolation, however, in the fact that no one expects the student to believe that there are actual lotus-like objects somewhere in or around the body. The *chakras* as they are conceived are none other than *yantras*—mystical diagrams to help one meditate—and students are regularly guided by their gurus in the visualization of the diagrams in their various colours and shapes, a whole geometry of concentration. Like Swami Gnaneswarananda, most everybody involved with *laya-yoga* agrees that the idea of a sleeping serpent is a metaphor and 'the lotuses we have been speaking of are symbolic'.

After that, however, there is considerable disharmony and speculation, relating to where the centres and the serpent are in relation to the body we can see and feel. After all, an attractive aspect of Tantra is its assertion that the body matters, that it is not just something to be rushed away from into *nirvana*. The arguments focus on whether these mystic organs are properly physical, like the feelings of heat and excitation they can produce, or whether they are a mixture of the physical and something subtler, or whether they exist on some separate plane altogether, called 'subtle' or 'etheric'. The only agreement is that they are *not* spirit as such, because spirit lies beyond—above the crown of the head, as it were.

The 'physicalists', if one can call them that, tend to be people who want to reconcile an ancient Hindu theory with modern Western anatomy and physiology. For them, the *chakras* can be correlated with nerve plexuses, ductless glands, or other significant observable parts of the body. Such observers consequently make the following straight identifications:

muladhara-chakra	the gonads
svadhisthana	the adrenals
manipura	the pancreas
anahata	the thymus
vishuddha	the thyroid
ajna	the pituitary
sahasrara	the pineal

If the *nadis*, which Tantric speculators counted in their thousands, are then a Hindu approximation to the nervous system, then the *chakras* are more or less glandular. The *kundalini* snake could then be some kind of integrative process operating on the nerves of the spinal column, a process in principle capable of being investigated and understood by Western scientists, and bringing nervous system and glandular systems into a fuller unity, while also preparing the way for higher consciousness. Certainly, it seems entirely reasonable that the ancient Tantric sages with their interest in bodies might examine corpses and speculate on internal processes, creating as they went along a cartography of the inner person. It is an attractive theory, partly because it makes the whole subject yet another proof of the wisdom of the East, brings it in line with the wisdom of the West, and enables friendly sceptics to cope with an otherwise silly-looking piece of medievalism. What is more, it is highly plausible, because the *nadis* are a lot like a proto-nervous system, and the *chakras* are astonishingly close to the glands.

More fully supported among enthusiasts for the *chakras*, however, is the view that all this is fair enough, but the Tantric system is greatly superior to what Western medical science understands about the body. In this view there is certainly a correspondence between, for example, *chakras* and glands, but the two are not identical. Glands belong in the gross physical body, while the *chakras* (and the *nadis*, and *kundalini*) belong in the subtle physical body. Swami Gnaneswarananda might content himself with saying that 'these symbols of lotuses stand for the different stages through which the soul passes on its journey towards infinite Perfection . . . are therefore *different stages of consciousness*', but Georg Feuerstein speaks for the generality of this group of 'correlationists' when he says:

The *cakras* have repeatedly been identified with the nerve plexi of the body, but these can at best be understood as correlated phenomena or physiological analogies . . . They [the *chakras*] are to be conceived of as force centres in the subtle or mind 'field' interlocked with and interpenetrating the physical body. However, it is still a moot question whether or not the *cakras* are essential components of the subtle body of all beings or are called into existence only by the higher practice of Yoga. In the *Bhairavī-Dīkṣā* . . . the *cakras* are pronounced to be created as a result of the ascent of the serpent fire and thus are held not to exist in the ordinary human being.[42]

Here we encounter Tantric élitism: the view that only special people with a special set of techniques can have special benefits. This suggestion that the *chakras* are created by mystical effort is a minority view, however, even among the members of the third group—the 'occultists', East and West, who do not consider the nervous system or the glands of any real significance. For them, the *chakras*, *nadis*, and *kundalini* belong on the subtle level of matter alone, not on the gross level of the body. For them, the Tantric experimenters who created the theory and practice of *laya-yoga* have had access to a 'science' that is a higher truth than any so far, or likely to be, apprehended by Western science and medicine.

Peter Rendel speaks from this position when he says: 'In order to understand the chakras or vital force centres and how they relate to each other, one must first begin by studying how the essential polarities of Spirit and Matter came into existence.'[43] He assumes that we can in fact know this, and proceeds to discuss 'our own true Eternal Self', levels of distinction of 'the finer from the grosser', the Qabalah, Hermeticism, alchemy, astrology, 'the occult anatomy of man', polarities like the Chinese yin and yang, rhythms and cycles of life which he calls 'the Tattwic Tides', 'the four pole magnet' and other ideas drawn from Eastern and Western occultism. As with all such approaches, one does not start from proof but with a leap of faith. The terminology used and the assumptions made are not open either to philosophical discussion or to scientific assessment. Whatever the merits of occultism and its rich symbolic life, it operates in the religious rather than the scientific sphere. Either you believe, or you do not.

Ultimately, therefore, what one makes of *chakra* and *kundalini* appears to depend upon personality and inclination. If one wishes to stay in the world of the everyday and of scientific caution, one favours the nerves-and-glands explanation, plus something science does not yet understand but *could* understand. If one believes that Western science is still a long way short of understanding the subtleties of the physical world, then one accepts the subtler-grosser correlation, which has the merit of being close to the traditional Hindu position. If one is dubious about Western science and willing to dismiss it as a stumbling materialist procedure, and if one also inclines towards the view that there is in the world a kind of hidden brotherhood of Those Who Know, then one prefers the wholly subtle position and its synthesis of ideas from a variety of occult backgrounds. Finally, if one is unsure, one simply swings around among the three positions, depending upon the company one keeps at any particular time—including now and again dismissing the whole thing as pretentious nonsense.

What one cannot do, of course, in all honesty is dismiss the subject as pretentious nonsense. However described and explained, the picture of *chakras* and *kundalini* relates to something vigorous and at least subjectively real and quite probably objectively real as well. In practice, whatever the sleeping serpent is, it should not be forced into wakefulness, but rather as Swami Satchidananda puts it, in his symbolic language: 'You don't need to set fire to the snake. Instead, the gentle warmth goes there and says, "He seems to be doing well, you can just look up now." This method is much safer than forcing. It may take a little longer, but that doesn't matter. The longer road is the safer one. This way you are well prepared for the power. When it wakes up, you become a wonderful instrument.'[44]

Or, to give Georg Feuerstein the last word: 'No school of Yoga has been subjected to graver misunderstanding and greater hostility from uninformed critics, both in India and in the West, than *Kundalini-yoga*. True enough, its principles and practices are difficult to understand, though they possibly hold the key to many of the problems with which contemporary psychologists and biologists are battling. No field of research on Yoga seems to hold out a better prospect of yielding real core information about man, which is so wanting today.'[45]

In this, he and Basham appear to agree. The subject cries out for serious research.

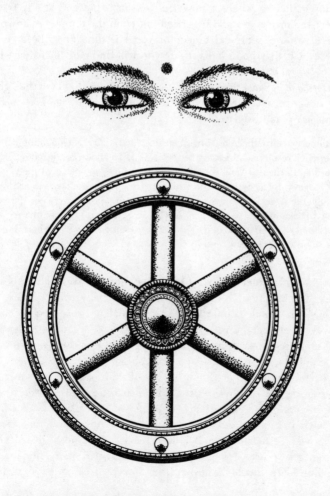

9. DARSHANA

In any gathering where a powerful person is present, at any festival where the image of a god is carried out from the temple, in any place where some exceptional object or force is thought to be at work, wherever it may be in India, there you will find individuals who have come 'to take darshan'.

Darshana in Sanskrit is simply 'seeing' or 'viewing', but in the sight or the view everything changes. As the 15th edition of the *Encyclopaedia Britannica* puts it, *darshana* is

in Hindu worship, the beholding of an auspicious deity, person, or object. The experience results in a blessing of the viewer. The boon conferred may differ according to the deity and the circumstances, time, and place, of the viewing. The *rathayātrās* (car festivals), in which images of gods are taken in procession through the streets, enable even those who in former days were not allowed to enter the temple to have *darśana* of the deity. *Darśana* (the bestowing of an opportunity to see) is also imparted by a guru (spiritual leader) to his followers, by a ruler to his subjects, and by the objects of veneration such as pilgrimage shrines to its [*sic*] visitors.

Although neither the word nor the concept is well known beyond India, the practice is common enough in many other places. The enthusiasm which people have to see (and possibly also to touch, however fleetingly) a member of the British royal family has a strong dash of *darshana* to it, as do the spontaneous eruptions among young people in the presence of a favoured pop star. The idea is ancient, part of the voodoo-like substratum of Hinduism; it presupposes some kind of transference of a more or less medicinal nature from the revered person-cum-object to the viewer. Anthropologists have found almost everywhere in the world a belief that numinous beings and objects give off power or radiation (and indeed need some kind of insulation to prevent that power being wasted). Thus, a deified ruler's feet may not be allowed to touch the ground, or a revered object is wrapped up except for display on special occasions. A common (though controversial word among anthropologists for this power is *mana*, a Melanesian term for inherent sacredness. While 'numinous' itself comes from the Latin *numen*, a quality that inspires religious awe. People go on pilgrimage because of *darshana*-related beliefs, and expectations of cures in places like Lourdes or at the touch of a king date back to a time when the whole human race apparently believed in degrees of numinous power all around them—some greater, some lessor, some kinder, some more malign. Officially, in today's more or less 'educated' world, this kind of animistic and magical view is confined to more 'primitive' peoples and minds, and permissible only among small children and in works of fantasy; it has been banished, at least on the surface, but there is plenty of evidence in popular responses to queens and popes, swamis, and saints that the belief lives on and is widespread.

This kind of *darshana* matters in yoga because all over India gurus do give *darshana* to their followers, and even people who do not particularly believe in Guru A or Swami B will linger at his meetings in case some personal benefit reaches them. Western occultists can relate this 'radiation' to the aura, to energies and vibrations. Western scientists will be cautious or sceptical, but the prima facie evidence of faith healing and so-called miracle cures suggests that caution is the wiser course here. Simply labelling certain responses 'psychosomatic' is not very helpful in such matters, because we need to know just how one person's psyche can have a potent influence over somebody else's soma. If some kind of force passed between them, then we should know about it. If it did not, but still the other's presence prompted a cure, we should know about that too. Either way, to ignore such phenomena as *darshana* and faith healing is itself hardly scientific.

This is the superficially more sensational of the two meanings of *darshana*. It is not, however, necessarily the more significant in the long run. The second meaning is much more intellectual and philosophical, but by no means dry and dull, and quite capable of revolutionizing our ideas of what 'reality' is.

Knowledge has always been venerated in India, whether it is the lesser knowledge of things in the world or the greater knowledge of transcendental reality. Classically speaking, knowledge could be acquired from three sources: one's own perceptions, one's own logical inferences, and the traditions around us that help shape our perceptions and inferences. However, nothing in this contingent world is complete or perfect, so knowledge in that world is naturally incomplete and imperfect. This fact was particularly well appreciated by the rigorous and pessimistic Jains with their *syadvada* or 'theory of maybe'. As Hiriyanna puts it:

It signifies that the universe can be looked at from many points of view, and that each view-point yields a different conclusion (anekanta). The nature of reality is expressed completely by none of them, for in its concrete richness it admits all predicates. Every proposition is therefore in strictness only conditional. Absolute affirmation and absolute negation are both erroneous. The Jains illustrate this position by means of the story of a number of blind people examining an elephant and arriving at varying conclusions regarding its form while in truth each observer has got at only a part of it. The doctrine indicates extreme caution and signifies an anxiety to avoid all dogma in defining the nature of reality.[46]

To the Jains—however rigidly they in fact worked out their own system and followed it—reality is too baffling for absolute description, and to make their point they offered a 'seven-fold formula' to prove it:

1. Maybe it is.
2. Maybe it is not.
3. Maybe it is and is not.
4. Maybe it is inexpressible.
5. Maybe it is and is inexpressible.
6. Maybe it is not and is inexpressible.
7. Maybe it is and is not and is inexpressible.

In modern Western terms, the Jains were proposing 'models' of reality: perhaps the world is like X, or imagine that the cosmos is Y, or let us agree that the universe is not (like) Z. Whether such comparisons were models or metaphors, however, they have been popular in India, both inside Hinduism and as part of the heterodox systems of the Jains and the Buddhists. There were different darshanas—'viewpoints' or 'visions' or 'frames of reference'—available of how reality could be structured, but always with the proviso that no picture could ever be large and clear enough, no system profound enough, to fit the totality. In the West we are only now coming to terms with the idea that optional models can be created to help us understand things; it is chastening to learn that they have been available in the East for an unknown number of centuries. From time to time, of course, individual theorists have felt that they knew the ultimate truth (the Buddha appears to have been one), but, by and large, sadhus and sages have been content to smile and say that reality is a cart-wheel: we live on the rim and wish to go to the centre. Consequently, we follow a single, straight spoke to get there. Each spoke is different: a different path (marga), technology (yoga) or discipline (sadhana), but all ultimately leading to the same place.

Moving on from discussion of the Jains and their theory of maybe, Hiriyanna talks about the orthodox Hindu darshana, 'which literally means "sight", and may be taken to indicate that what the Indians aspired after in philosophy was not a mediated knowledge of the ultimate truth but a direct vision of it. The word in that case would express what is a distinguishing feature of Indian philosophy in general—its insistence that one should not rest content with a mere intellectual conviction but should aim at transforming such conviction into direct experience.'[47] Here, philosophic *darshana* meets the *darshana* of a guru or a god: having thought his way through the logic of a system—having followed the spoke of the wheel from the rim to the hub—the philosopher seeks and is rewarded with direct unmediated knowledge, no longer the knowledge of books and debate, but a transcendental appreciation of, and immersion in, the essence of the Real.

As Alain Daniélou points out:

> according to their own logic and means of proof, some of the 'points of view' (*darśana*) must be atheistic, others pantheistic, others deistic, moralistic, mystical. Yet we should not hastily conclude that these are the conflicting beliefs of philosophers. They are only the logical conclusions drawn from the premises and reached through the methods acceptable for each approach, each 'point of view'. Each one is real within its own field and aims towards the utmost limit of the reach of our faculties in a particular direction. The builders of the 'points of view' are not spoken of as thinkers or prophets but as seers (*ṛṣi*).[48]

Thus, you adopt a guru and a *sadhana* and follow the instructions of the guru and the rules of the *sadhana*. This places you upon the spoke, along which you travel with steady determination, until the hub is reached. Even arriving at the hub you will see it differently from another person at the end of another spoke, but it is the same hub.

Out of all the *darshanas* that have arisen in India, classical Hinduism recognizes six core systems, the *Shaddarshanas* ('The Six Points of View'). They operate in pairs, and cover a wide range of intellectual interests as follows:

1. The system of logic called *Nyaya* ('analysis'), linked with:
2. The system of physics or natural philosophy called *Vaisheshika* ('individual characteristics').
3. The system of cosmology called *Sankhya* ('numbers'), linked with:
4. The system of integration called *Yoga* ('union').
5. The system of Vedic textual study called *Mimamsa* ('inquiry'), linked with:
6. The system of salvationist philosophy called *Vedanta* ('the end, goal, or conclusion of the Vedas').

Hinduism being Hinduism, this neat set of *darshanas* is more of a tidy intellectual scheme than a widely appreciated aid. The systems have odd relations the one with the other, as well as with other systems not conceived as orthodox and classical. Thus, *Vaisheshika* is remarkable for its theory of atoms, shared with Jain philosophy and on a par with the classical atomic theory of the Greeks. Similarly, *Sankhya* has strong historical and attitudinal links with Buddhism, of which it may well have been a direct predecessor; neither system treats divinity as centrally important, and yet *Sankhya* also figures strongly in the *Gita*, which is a theistic treatise. *Nyaya*-cum-*Vaisheshika* was in fact classical India's system of logic and natural science, little concerned with escape from the wheel of life and death. *Sankhya*-cum-*Yoga* was a system of harmonizing the human microcosm with the universal macrocosm, through intellectual understanding (*buddhi*) and a clear-cut regime of physical and mental behaviour (Patanjali's *ashthanga-yoga*), and a rival to the Buddha's *ashthangika-marga*. *Mimamsa*-cum-*Vedanta* were a brahminical playground of textual authoritarianism combined with the speculation of the *Upanishads*. Vedanta and Yoga are the two most vigorous movements today, have enormously cross-fertilized each other while being influenced in all sorts of ways by non-Vedic movements like Buddhism, Tantrism and Bhaktism—and the result is the easy-come-easy-go potpourri of ecumenical thinking so common in India today and in yoga circles around the world.

Not that that is necessarily a bad thing, as long as the mélange of terminologies can be separated out. The idea of *darshana* allows for, as it were, all sorts of blends and 'super-darshanas', such as Sri Aurobindo's Integral Yoga. The only danger is that without a certain amount of straightforward scholarly analysis the mass of ancient, medieval, and modern systems will become, in interested people's heads, a mess of vaguely understood and misunderstood terms. Given that gurus are a common phenomenon and that what they have learned from *their* gurus may be a synthesis of blends of hybrid systems dating back over centuries, then the buyer should sometimes beware. Language complicates the issue, because what may be clear enough to Hindu exponents of this or that yoga may not be clear when rendered into English or when the original terms are embedded in English. Thus, there are at least four separate main terms often translated as 'liberation' or 'enlightenment': *moksha, mukti, kaivalya,* and *nirvana*. They relate to different *darshanas*, and need to be watched. Sometimes they are interchangeable; at other times they are not.

The concept of *darshana* can be marvellously broad-minded and cosmopolitan, or it can be a mishmash of hazily understood syncretic terms and techniques. In the West today, much like India's spiritual bazaars over the centuries, a kind of smorgasbord style has developed that is often perilously close to dilettantism: a little hatha-yoga today, some Zen next week, a touch of Tantra here, a modicum of Tai-chi-chuan there. Traditionally, though, a *darshana* has had its own special shape, belonging to a group with a verifiable identity; new gurus could alter the shape and the tradition, but the historical links remained, legitimate spokes to the wheel of philosophical and religious effort. Nowadays, given the global melting pot and the argument that everybody should be free to do his or her own thing (and go to heaven or hell their own various ways) the liberating value of a concept like this can begin to look like licence and excess—on the part of both the mini-gurus and the kinds of laid-back disciples that Gita Mehta describes in *Karma Cola*. No one has yet captured better the horror and the humour of instant pop mysticism:

The next day I went off to hear God's morning discourse. God sat in a cushioned swivel chair with a blue denim hat on his head and spoke about the revolution. As the discourse gathered momentum it became clear that God was an intellectual snob. He dropped only the heaviest names. Jesus. Marx. Mahavira. And Fritz Perls. His two-thousand-odd devotees, inhaled, writhed or listened in an ecstasy of *being*.

Present in the gathering were several Japanese and Korean disciples who spoke no English. They sat in the early morning sunlight staring at God with beatific smiles, the envy of their occidental brothers.

'They can hear with their hearts. There are no words to stand between them and God's pure energy. They can be one with him.'

'Did you feel God's aura? Did you get a hit off the energy?'

'It's all words, words, words,' says Essex with a deep sigh. 'Why can't you just sit here with us and BE? Gradually our energies will overlap and we will understand each other without speaking.'

California nods assent.

'Yeah. You know, lady, you should join in some of our meditations. You could learn to be silent and exist. You look like you need it. To be. It's really a terrific high.'

California winks archly. 'It's better than coming.'

Doubtless. Doubtless. But how will they handle going?[49]

Gita Mehta does not identify the guru-God or his followers, who had in fact swapped their Western names for Sanskrit labels given to them by their guru. Identification, however, is not particularly important. The coming together of eager but befuddled Westerners with equally eager Eastern spiritual guides is now an established part of the late twentieth century. Western guides in Eastern garb are also arising and calling themselves avatars and buddhas, while Eastern gurus in the West offer everybody a new world or the old world renewed through mystic waves of energy. In due course the sociology of this process will be written, describing the nature of the Beatles' relationship with Maharishi Mahesh Yogi, providing an objective account of whether the Ananda Marga sect were actually murderers and explaining why Bhagwan Shree Rajneesh left India, set up Rajneeshpuram in Oregon, and at length came to denounce some of his own leading disciples as thieves and murderers.

There is nothing specially new about this. It has been happening inside India for centuries. The only 'new' element is that the confusions of gurudom, godmen, and spiritual paths have burst the bounds of the Subcontinent. Where old syntheses, re-alignments, successes, and failures once occurred only among the Hindus, Buddhists, and Jains (with a bit of help now and again from Muslims and Christians in India), they are now part and parcel of the global melange. From scholar to hippie, from theologian to theosophist, from scientist to occultist, from fitness freak to physician, from Radhakrishnan and Aurobindo in the East to Bede Griffiths and Fritzhof Capra in the West, the ways from rim to hub of the cosmic wheel are open to all sorts of new arrangements, interpretations, and alignments. 'Make straight the way of the Lord,' is no longer necessarily an applicable command. One can be a Zen-Sufi, a Christian Yogi, a mystical physicist, a scientific Vedantist . . .

There are of course still many tightly structured *sadhanas* with their traditional *darshanas* virtually intact, in India and elsewhere. They offer straight paths, traditional spokes from rim to hub, and often insist, in a fundamentalist way, that their route is the only true route, and their vision the only true vision. There are also new systems and visions being formed in the creative swirl of 'the Aquarian Age', some rather casual and temporary, others with the prospect of a certain permanence. And thirdly, there are many part-*darshanas*, bits and pieces of this and that stitched together, fragments of the old childhood religions tacked onto shards of newly adopted and unevenly understood substitutes. This latter is typical of times of rapid change, in which many people are uncomfortably adrift among too many options.

We live in an interesting but perilous time. Cultures now meet that in the past had little to do with each other, and once used de-contamination rituals when they did chance to meet. Hard-liners from every background offer their stiff certainties to the insecure and the inquisitive from every other background. The vast worldviews of Buddhism, Christianity, Hinduism, and Islam—no longer safe in their geographical and mental cocoons—confront each other in some confusion, and are all at risk from the success of Western science and technology with their materialist slant. It is understandable that many people will take some sort of refuge in infantilism—back to the mother's milk of a fundamentalist system. Others take fright at the totalitarian quality of the traditional scriptures. Others still are willing to dabble in drugs and hallucination, eager to transcend the confusion. However, though the scale is new, there is nothing specially new in the phenomenon itself. The Buddha would have recognized it.

In this rich, chaotic situation the concept of *darshana* could be a valuable aid. It is as ancient as the Jains and yet can handle the relativity of Einstein. It insists that in this world there are no absolutes of truth available to the Chosen Few, or to the masses If They Would Only Listen. It also proposes that it is not possible to talk in ordinary everyday language about what lies beyond ordinary everyday language.

What is available, however, can be either mental flux or mental discipline. It is necessary to adopt some kind of working frame of reference, from the very rigid to the very flexible, but in terms of human maturity, a flexible, open-eyed system whose limits one appreciates is a saner, safer bet. As the philosopher of science Karl Popper might put it, there are no absolutes here, only more or less, better or worse relative positions.

That is all we have. The choice lies between blundering around in the maya of existence, or accepting a rigid and limited way of thinking that will get us through our days, or with due care and attention building a strong but subtle personal *darshana*, weighing the options with care. Such a system could evolve as we evolve. Structures and frames of any kind are like crutches in a universe where everyone is relatively disabled. Your crutches may be devotionally adjusted, linked with selfless service, tied to the intellect; they might require their symbolism in terms of Christ or Krishna, they might be theosophical and occult or free-thinking and scientific, socialist or capitalist, a blend of a number of ideologies more or less consciously worked out. There could even be short-term *sadhanas* and *darshanas*, demanding, say, celibacy or vegetarianism, or allowing free love and doing one's own thing. They would not have a cast-iron guarantee built into any of them, because there are no such guarantees in this world. The only fact appears to be that the materials out of which one can build one's personal philosophy are lying all around.

This, however, is only another *darshana*, and no god was present—as far as I know—when it was committed to paper.

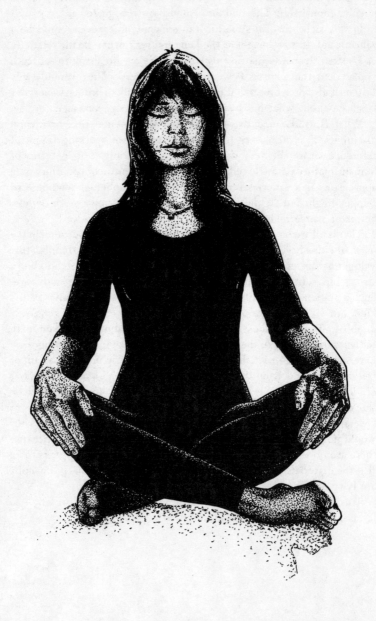

10. DHYANA

'There was a monkey,' says Swami Vivekananda, 'restless by his own nature, as all monkeys are. As if that were not enough, someone made him drink freely of wine, so that he became still more restless. Then a scorpion stung him. When a man is stung by a scorpion he jumps about for a whole day: so the poor monkey found his condition worse than ever. To complete his misery a demon entered into him. What language can describe the uncontrollable restlessness of that monkey?

'The human mind is like that monkey, incessantly active by its own nature: then it becomes drunk with the wine of desire, thus increasing its turbulence. After desire takes possession comes the sting of the scorpion of jealousy at the success of others, and last of all the demon of pride enters the mind, making it think itself of all importance. How hard to control such a mind!'[50]

Vivekananda drew this analogy of mind with monkey while describing and discussing the eight limbs of Patanjali's yoga. Elsewhere he used that other favourite of yoga teachers, mind as a disturbed lake or pond. That is the analogy with which Patanjali himself begins when he says that the practice of his yoga is *chittavritti-nirodhah*, 'the stilling of the ripples of the mind'. Patanjali's text is a classic of systematizing and condensing, one of the world's earliest self-improvement courses, harsh and alien to many Westerners but of great importance in the history of humanity's attempts, as it were, to rise above itself. His system and the systems of Gautama the Buddha and other practical mystics in India and elsewhere broadly agree about misery and the mind, and from their various recommendations one can distil the following eight elements in a *sadhana* or course of spiritual discipline:

1. Some kind of general ethical preparation.
2. A peaceful attitude in a peaceful setting.
3. A firm, comfortable and unstrained position, usually seated.
4. Steadiness, including steady breathing.

5. A sense of detachment; a willingness to be apart and alone.
6. The stilling of the body and a retreat from its demands.
7. Focusing or concentrating the mind into one-pointedness.
8. The stilling of the mind and a retreat from thought.

This is the basic pattern of self-preparation certainly for Indian mysticism if not for mysticism at large. People and groups differ as to details (some of which are considered very important details) but probably agree on the broad picture. This picture leaves out of consideration the content of the ethical preparation, just how peaceful peaceful should be (does it mean pacifism?), what form the breathing should take, how detached detached should be, whether retreating from the body's demands means self-starvation, celibacy, etc., and a variety of other points that I do not propose to consider here. In India, however, one may add, the preparations have tended to be severe rather than gentle, ascetic rather than domestic, and religious rather than secular, although gentle and domestic and secular variants have all existed. Generally, to aid in the aspirant's detachment and concentration, various focusing devices have traditionally been made available to Indians, and these are:

1. *murti*: an image (usually of a god)
2. *mantra*: a 'thought-form' expressed as sound
3. *japa*: the repetition of sounds
4. *mudra*: a gesture or 'seal', usually of the hand(s)
5. *yantra*: a more or less complex geometric diagram
6. *asana*: a stylized seated position or bodily pose

All of these are aids to *dhyana*, which Patanjali presents as the seventh of the eight limbs or elements in his system. This word is most commonly translated into English as 'meditation', but is also sometimes rendered as 'mental concentration' and as 'contemplation', particularly of a religious kind. It is and is not these things. It derives from *dhyai* which means 'to think' in the sense of reflecting, of being attentive and, most significantly, of being absorbed. It refers to a special kind of inner-directedness. It is not what one does in a market-place or on the field of battle, but the assumption is that if in calm seclusion one has practised *dhyana* alongside the other requirements of one's 'spiritual' discipline, then it could be sustained on a battlefield and can certainly help in the clamour of life. And the reason for that is *dhyana*'s capacity to attune us to the great stillness at the heart of all the bustle and mayhem of life.

The West has its own systems of religious contemplation, its own monastic rules and traditions of mystic communion. These have a lot in common with yoga and other Indian *sadhanas*, but differ from them in being less of a technology of self-realization. They are not as firmly mapped out, they do not offer the same guarantees, nor do they strive after a cessation of thought and what suspiciously resembles oblivion. More like the Hindu *bhakti* cults, their aim is the Beatific Vision—looking directly on the face of God. In the various yogas, however, and that includes *bhakti-yoga*, you have a programmatic ladder to climb, and the rungs have supported many feet before yours. The rungs are usually neatly labelled too. Confusingly, however, the yogas differ about what you meet at the top of the ladders: Krishna waiting with arms to enfold you, the divine union of Shiva and Shakti, the approving nod of a remote Lord Ishwara, a smiling Buddha in the Pure Land of the West, or *nirvana* ('the blowing out') and *kaivalya* ('isolation').

Dhyana is a word and concept that has travelled far. In Pali, a classical language of the Buddhists, it is *jhana*, in which form it went to China and became *ch'an*, in which form it went further, to Japan, and became *zen*. It has therefore exerted an enormous influence on several of the major civilizations of the earth and on innumerable people within those civilizations. That surely singles it out as a significant subject in its own right, even if, say, yoga or Buddhism alone did not merit much study. Psychologists, neurologists, and chemists should all be interested in it, quite apart from philosophers and mystics. It is, after all, one of the very few concepts which suggests that we can do more with the mind than simply run the body, observe our surroundings, and make plans.

How does one start to meditate, continue meditating, and recognize that one has achieved something by meditating? And what, at the end of the day, has been going on?

'The first lesson,' says Vivekananda, 'is to sit for some time and let the mind run on. The mind is bubbling up all the time. It is like that monkey jumping about. Let the monkey jump as much as he can: you simply wait and watch. Knowledge is power, says the proverb, and that is true. Until you know what the mind is doing you cannot control it. Give it the rein; many hideous thoughts will come into it; you will be astonished that it was possible for you to think such thoughts. But you will find that each day the mind's vagaries are becoming less and less violent, that each day it is becoming calmer.'[51]

His fellow Vedantist Swami Ashokananda makes a similar point, but moving the student one stage further: 'Here is a psychological truth, wonderfully encouraging and helpful but often forgotten by spiritual aspirants. Once a man came to Shri Ramakrishna, saying, "I cannot control my mind—I don't know how". The Master, astonished, said,

"Why do you not practise *abhyasa-yoga*?" Bringing the mind back again and again to the thought of God—that is what *abhyasa-yoga* means . . . Does it matter very much if the mind wanders in the beginning, so long as you bring it back to Him?'[52] Or to the *murti*, the *mantra*, the *yantra* or whatever other aid or focus you are using.

It is clear from these suggestions that people who want to gain from meditation are in for a long haul—in traditional terms. And yet out of the self-same India in which Ramakrishna lived and taught has come in recent years, from Rishikesh in the Himalayas, a recipe for 'transcendental meditation' that is offered to the world for a measure of money and as a kind of psychic analogue to instant coffee and fast food. Maharishi Mahesh Yogi has cut through the fabric of the ages and presented us with a form of inner-directedness that fits in rather well with the hectic, action-packed life of the Western and Westernizing world. Set aside a little time each day for your mantra, he proposes, and it will do you good. If enough people follow suit, it could change the world. As a simple merchandizing exercise, TM is a brilliant achievement—a truly radical departure in the history of mysticism anywhere and anywhen.

And it has a beneficial effect. Scientific investigation has demonstrated that TM calms the people who engage in it, in particular increasing the flow of alpha waves in the brain, a factor which has also been recorded with Zen monks in Japan. Something comparable appears, therefore, to be happening in the truncated and trendy approach of the Maharishi and in the traditional approach of Zen Buddhism. That itself should be enough to give us pause. Quite apart from climbing to the heights of mysticism's Everest, it seems clear that even a minimal involvement with the simple techniques of yogic meditation has a beneficial effect, and has a future in therapeutic work as well as in private programmes of self-development.

That, however, is only the threshold stage. Yogis, sufis, saints, and mystics have all described their meditational adventures in terms of a kind of inner space or world where things happen once the monkey of the superficial world has been somewhat tranquillized. There is the curious inner sound of the 'unstruck bell', and there is the celebrated or notorious 'inner light' that occultists often talk about. There may be voices along the way that are disturbingly like the voices that schizophrenics hear, or that prophets have responded to. There is also the possibility of visions, dream-like on the mindscape, but hallucinations when they are cast upon the screen of the world. The literature of saints and seekers abounds with accounts of such phenomena, often described in the fantasy language of myth. What is one to make of such happenings? Are they to be taken literally or metaphorically? Are they facts as such, or are they analogical experiences, ways of seeing the unseeable and hearing the unhearable?

It is a vexed question. There are people who treat them as more or less symbolic and figurative. There are other people who believe that such inner events are more real than the sounds and sights of the outer world. And there are people who conceive of other planes of existence where other beings live and move—and can be contacted in the still journeyings of the mind.

One's background or worldview evidently affects the issue. When people travel into territory like this, what they 'see' and 'hear' is likely to conform to what they expect to see and hear. Thus, a Hindu in deep meditation might meet Krishna or Kali, while a Christian could meet Christ, the Virgin Mary or a favoured saint. A spiritualist-occultist could well encounter archangelic beings, and—who knows?—an enthusiast for Unidentified Flying Objects might meet beings from a UFO. In the vocabulary of Carl Gustav Jung, all these would be potent variants of the 'archetypes' in our collective unconscious, turned into 'archetypal images' that make sense in terms of our inheritance of specific religions and structures of belief and myth. In his view, intriguingly, all such manifestations are 'psychologically' real.

If one is indeed doing what Patanjali supposed, clearing the mind while wrapt in meditation, then it should come as no surprise that there are layers upon layers to be cleared. All sorts of sights, sounds, personalities, entities, visionary encounters, and galvanizing images might surface along the way. After all, they are common enough in our dreams and in the heritage of our race, and must therefore be just as much a part of the monkey's hopping and jumping as our ordinary sense impressions and everday tangle of thoughts.

They could of course be marvellously distracting too. If, for example, one met a numinous being somewhere in the reaches of the mind, such a personality—noble or nasty—might seem (be?) very impressive indeed. One might suppose that one was talking to (and walking with) God, and such experiences can occur without the stable platform of meditation. The world is full of people who have heard voices and seen visions, and responded to them in various ways. At one end of the continuum, religions have been founded by them; at the other end of the continuum, mental hospitals are full of them. It is by no means an unusual phenomenon, and there is no reason to suppose that mythic inner experiences are confined to 'messiahs' on the one hand and 'mad people' on the other. It is not therefore so important that one has such experiences. From the point of view of yogic meditation it is much

more important that one is not de-railed by them, or by the curious
siddhis ('powers') that are listed (by people like Patanjali) as possibly
accompanying them.

The issue is complicated by our very ignorance. Science cannot prove
categorically that disembodied entities do not exist, nor can occultism
demonstrate conclusively to science that they do. And even if one had
stronger evidence than we have that spiritual voyagers can encounter
strange events and beings, we would still need a theory to help us
account for such things. 'Realness' in such a subtle mind-world is
clearly not the same as the 'realness' of everyday sticks and stones,
people and places. And the area of interplay between the two worlds is
by no means clear. No one has yet said the last word on ghosts and
poltergeists, divine visions and voices, spirit contacts and table
rappings, dowsing and supernatural powers, possession and clairvoy-
ance. We may take sides, but that is currently all we do in the face of a
formidable mass of human experience that does not fit neatly into any
worldviews that we have—scientific, occult, or religious. We do not
yet have a theory broad and flexible enough to house what one half of
the human race claims happens to it, and that the other half mocks.

The issue is also complicated by the fact that mystics do not take too
seriously the distinction between what is 'spiritually' real and what is
'physically' real, except to state or imply that the higher reality of
mysticism is a truer appreciation of what is than the lower state in which
we normally live. To talk about the higher state, they have been
accustomed to use metaphors, and appear to have been accustomed to
other people taking their symbolic pictures as reality. Again, the mind is
a funny place, and a dream can seem very real. One person's
hallucination is another person's solid fact, and we are left with the
Buddha's smile at the end of all the speculation.

According to the majority of yogis and mystics, there is no talking
about, or seeing, or hearing the ultimate. It lies beyond phenomena—
both external and internal—and the goal of serious meditation is to take
you at least to the threshold of the Beyond, at least for a moment or two,
and perhaps longer if you persevere.

Thus, if the way is being properly followed, according to the
traditions, then an opening-up will occur, and something from
somewhere else will flood in . . . There, a metaphor again: the flooding
in of water or of light . . . God is encountered if you want God, or the
ineffable Atman-Brahman if you want that, or the Void of Nothingness
if that is your preference and you like something described negatively
although it lies beyond both positive and negative. Zen has its own stark
metaphors for this ultimate condition, as Eugene Herrigel has pointed
out:

For the Zen Buddhist everything that exists, apart from man—animals and plants, stones, earth, air, fire, water—lives undemandingly from the center of being, without having left it or being able to leave it. If man, having strayed from this center, is to know security and innocence of existence as they live it . . . there is no alternative for him but a radical reversal. He must go back along the way whose thousand fears and tribulations have shown it to be a way of error, must slough off everything that promised to bring him to himself, renounce the seductive magic of a life lived on his own resources, and return home to the 'house of truth' which he wantonly left in order to chase phantoms when he was scarcely fledged. He must not 'become as a little child,' but like forest and rock, like flower and fruit, like wind and storm.[53]

Patanjali's aim, the stilling of the ripples of the mind, the cessation of thought, is a scary ambition, when one thinks about it. As indeed is seeking the Beatific Vision, or Cosmic Consciousness, or Union with God, or Oblivion, or Release, or any other of the metaphors. It is rather like that other favourite of the yogis, stopping the heartbeat and then duly starting it up again, of which there have been many convincing reports.

There is a great deal of the paranormal in yoga that cannot simply be wished or explained away. Possibly the most paranormal of all is the ineffable state called variously *samadhi* ('making it all one'), *nirvana* ('blowing it all out'), *mukti* ('release'), *moksha* ('liberation'), *ananda* ('bliss') and *kaivalya* ('isolated freedom'). It is claimed to be a condition available both during life and after death, and to be equated neither with life nor death as such. Too many people have been involved with it for too long for it to be a delusion, an illusion, or a lie. It has been reached. It is both attainable and sustainable, just as they say it is—and one can lose it again afterwards, just as they warn can happen.

But how can we characterize it, this goal of meditation in particular and yoga in general?

Push the findings of Western science as far as they will go, and we can say that meditation influences the electro-chemical activity of the brain, among other bodily responses. In doing so, it creates an altered state of consciousness not unlike the hypnotic state; the only problem here being that we do not know what consciousness is or what the hypnotic state is either. However, in terms that balance yoga with science respectably, we can add that after the body has been sufficiently stilled and sense impressions sufficiently distanced, the mind enters a condition of 'sensory deprivation', which is a most unusual state indeed. In this state, the mind has been slipped out of gear.

If, however, meditation has been combined, as it often is, with such other techniques as fasting, drug-taking, extreme isolation, and torture-like activities, the deprived state can be attended by bizarre hallucinations. It may also be attended by 'mystical' events of the kundalini type, more or less violent depending on the regime being followed, and rendering the totally withdrawn state intermittent rather than smoothly continuous.

Where the meditation has not been mixed with harsh regimes and chemical aids, or at a point when these have been dispensed with, the mind can, and does, become deeply tranquil, unresponsive to outside stimuli. Having had a longer or a shorter experience of this kind, dedicated individuals may, and often do, experience attitudinal changes, and these have traditionally been described in terms of an inflow of 'intuitive knowledge' in comparison with which worldly knowledge of even the highest kind is unreal—is, in fact, ignorance. The result of these changes is, in many cases, a person with greater detachment and spiritual-cum-philosophical strength. Such a person, however, is not necessarily home and dry at such a stage, because he or she can be sucked back by the blandishments of *maya*, and there is ample evidence of this happening to even the most revered of rishis.

At the limits of meditative awareness, science, language and myth alike abandon the task of description and the experiencer appears to become more attuned to 'being' than 'doing'. A double focus occurs, so that such a person operates as it were with binocular vision, able to see in two 'worlds', simultaneously.

All of which concerns systematic exposure to the processes of meditation over a long period. It also suggests that, whatever the other 'vision', it is naturally available to the human race and is not just the province of a few God-touched people. It is in fact, according to many yogis, our natural condition. In a haphazard form, it appears to be available to all kinds of people, whether or not they would be regarded as spiritually respectable: the drug-taker (shaman or hedonist), the contemplative monk, the hippie living 'an alternative lifestyle', the soldier overcome in the midst of battle, an accident victim on the edge of apparent death, the yogi in a far place, the poet lost in reverie, the artist inspired, the dancer transported, and many others.

The essential difference between these longer or shorter snatches of the transcendental and the steady-state awareness of yoga lies in the sheer calculation of the yogi: you do this, you do that, you do the other, and in due course you have the experience, and you do it all some more (whatever it is you have been doing), and you have the experience for a longer time until in the end—all things being equal—you know and others know that you are 'a realized self'.

How you talk to other people about it (*if* you talk to other people about it) depends on how you and they have been conditioned to handle (or to fail to handle) such things. You can bring in God or the alpha rhythms, God *and* the alpha rhythms, or the Great Void, or anything else, but none of it matters. By definition all of this is conditioned. By definition, however you got there, nobody can talk about what lies at the end of *dhyana*'s rainbow.

By definition, if we could talk about it, it would not have been worth the effort expended getting there.

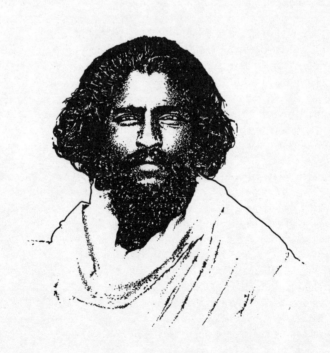

11. GURU and SHISHYA

'Swami Vishnu Devananda was the presiding guru at this symposium in Spain,' wrote Jane Thomson, yoga teacher and teacher trainer in Scotland, 'and I looked forward to seeing his outrageous personality again, no small reason being that he had the earliest and probably the strongest influence inclining me towards a certain yogic path. I remembered his favourite chant had always been "Be up and at it—pranayam, asan . . ." Whatever he wanted you doing, you did . . Certainly he wanted everybody "doing" (karma) all the time. I once heard someone referring to him as a bouncing orange dumpling filled with cosmic energy. It was as good a description as I could imagine.

'I did wonder if in the years since I had last seen him he had changed very much, particularly after his near-fatal accident six months previously. At the lecture following meditation it did not seem to be the case. There was Swamiji looking a little plumper, a little greyer, but still frolicking around on his huge orange cushion, laughing and snorting, whispering and shouting, wrapping part of his saffron attire around his head to make a turban—this to dress himself up in the part of a very serious holy man, strictly for our amusement. All culminating in a quake of giggles.

'Minutes later, unpredictable as ever, he gave the most inspiring lecture on the Origin of the Universe. There was no sky-larking now, only an excelsior figure urging us to surface up out of Maya, leap out of our cage of flesh, seek liberation. Then the full-lunged clarion call subsided to a leisurely relaxed conversation level as Swamiji tried to get through to us the "positive peace" of the yogic life.

'When I left the hall I felt as if I had been washed, mangled, ironed out straight and then left to waft whichever way the wind blew. As on previous occasions, I wished I had had the courage to ask, "Would the real - private - Swami Vishnu Devananda please make himself known, and reveal to us his state of belief at this moment?" Perhaps I couldn't because it seemed a form of guru-baiting. Apart from over-frenzied devotees, gurus have other problems. They are being watched and judged all the time, so in self-preservation they project an image. Sometimes the image is fashioned to inspire us with awe, sometimes it is humble enough to take one's breath away. It is one way to survive in the Here-and-Now.

'Then you wonder if they *have* survived. Have they become a little too attached to the offerings of the Here-and-Now? Aeroplanes, big cars, colour television, even getting your image on that television screen. Of course they had all been warned of the *siddhis*, but this magic, had they been prepared for *it*?'[54]

Jane Thomson represents a cool but involved Western position: profound interest in yoga and a concern at the same time about what she has labelled 'guruitis'. It is, she says, highly contagious when among the affected, yet one recovers very easily. As Gita Mehta waspishly makes clear in *Karma Cola*, however, not all Western enthusiasts recover so easily from whatever the contagion is; and, as traditional Hindu describers of the *guru-shishya* relationship have had it, recovery from this divine infection is exactly what one should not want. The *guru*, once found, is the way, the truth, and the life, utterly to be obeyed if success is to be achieved.

The word *guru* has a somewhat chequered past. Basically, it is a Sanskrit adjective meaning 'heavy', 'great', 'violent', 'severe', 'important', and 'venerable', all of which then serves to describe the brahmin teacher with whom the brahmin boy lived during his student days as a celibate *brahmachari*. The *Vedas* were the central object of study in the beginning, and it was only with the passage of the centuries that the word, still retaining its basic connotation of a teacher, any teacher, extended outward in socio-spiritual terms to include a master or mistress of any background, any caste, any system, who could teach a *sadhana* or spiritual discipline and around whom *shishyas* (or *chelas*) gathered. As late as the sixteenth century, numbers of *shishyas*—or, as the Punjabi dialect frames it, *Sikhs*—gathered around a tolerant and pacifist Guru Nanak, starting what has become a separate religion in India and across the world. The Sikhs had ten gurus in all, and then the accumulated power of those leaders was centred in one book of diverse scriptures, known thereafter as the Guru Granth Sahib. In the Golden Temple of Amritsar to this day, the Granth is treated like a person. I have watched it being wrapped in silken sheets, placed reverently in a palanquin, and carried across the single causeway from the Temple in its artificial lake to the Akal Takht building, where each night it 'sleeps' in a great bed. The *guru* therefore need not even be a person.

Yet all gurus have something of the divine in them, because it is believed that they have attained by their efforts or otherwise provide a fuller awareness of the divinity in and behind everything. They have surfaced up out of *maya*, and still deign to look down again, in order to help the rest of us. Or so the theory has it. Peter Brent wrote a whole book about the *guru* phenomenon. It is called *Godmen of India*, it was published in 1972, and in it he describes the virtual stereotype of the *Sad-guru*—the teacher of reality:

As a boy, he may be discovered to be religious, different from other children, as in the West artistically gifted children are different. Threatened with marriage, he will often refuse and leave home, to wander from one holy place to the next. Finally he will meet his fate—the Guru at whose feet he is destined to sit. Such a meeting may be early, he may leave and then return years later; or it may be after twenty years of searching. He remains with his Guru, he does all that is asked, he subjugates himself, he serves. When the Guru judges him ready, he receives his *diksha*, his initiation. He achieves longer and longer periods of samadhi, his holiness becomes apparent, people begin to speak of him with reverence. He may leave at this point and, while always retaining his connection with the Guru, set up in an ashram of his own; or he may stay and, when the old Guru dies, become the head and centre of his ashram. People come to him, he becomes famous and the ashram rich. Sooner or later, a new disciple of great potentiality will attach himself to him—the next Guru will have been found.[55]

So it has been proceeding for an unknown number of centuries in India, for at least three millennia in the longest unbroken apostolic succession anywhere in the world. The *Upanishads* are nearly that old, and they contain lists of gurus who were taught by gurus, back to the beginnings of Hindu time.

The relationship, however, is not always an easy one, and in it there has often been a touch of sado-masochism alongside the teacher-pupil devotion. B.K.S. Iyengar dedicates his successful and influential *Light on Yoga* (1966) to 'my Reverend Guruji, Samkhya-yoga-Sikhamani; Veda-kesari; Vedantavagisa; Nyayacharya; Mimamsa-ratna; Mimamsa-tirtha, Professor, Sriman, T Krishnamacharya of Mysore'. The dedication is accompanied by a photograph of this polymath of the spirit, and the dedication and picture serve, as it were, as Iyengar's own credentials. He belongs in the succession of the apostles of yoga, guru-blessed. His guru has all the Hindu spiritual equivalents of the Order of the British Empire and the Nobel Prize to prove it, for he is an authority in Sankhya and in Yoga, an expert on the *Vedas* and on Vedanta, knowledgeable in the logic of Nyaya and the ritual of Mimamsa. And yet, with disarming frankness, Iyengar can elsewhere write:

In my two years in Mysore, however, my guru hardly encouraged me nor did he explain to me the principles or the more subtle points of yoga. During the two years he did not teach me for more than forty days and never showed me how to get rid of the excruciating pains I had to endure. On the contrary he was often frighteningly fearful. Had circumstances not forced me I would never have gone on. People wanted me to teach them yoga and I was forced to practise. It was as simple as that. My interest was for the sake of earning my livelihood.'[56]

Once, in Bombay in the 1960s, I had a chat about *gurus* with Ramakrishna Alva, a friend who was also my wife's teacher of *bharata natyam*, one of the forms of classical Indian dancing. He was a gentle and affectionate man and he listened to me with a smile as I spoke rather disconsolately about the arrogance of certain *gurus*. When I finished, he said:

'Feel my head—here.'

I did as he asked, and felt a flattened area where the skin or the surface was strangely loose and mobile.

'What is that?' I asked. 'It isn't natural, is it?'

'Not at all. My guru used to hit me on the head with an iron bar. But you see, I had one thought only—to learn the dance—and he was the only way, so I had to take it.'

'Are a lot of gurus like that?'

'Oh yes. They treat their pupils like slaves. Not so bad now, but it used to be very bad. Ours is not yet a civilized country, Mr Tom.'

Ramakrishna and his wife Jayalakshmi were warm people, and yet they were strict disciplinarians. *Bharata natyam* is a demanding art form that has many of the features of a yoga, and its practitioners expect and get effort and concentration from their students. I used to sit at the side of the hall that they used, in the ex-palace of a rajah near Malabar Hill, to watch their techniques. It was riveting. There was no harshness or disdain, but the hard work got done, the students sweating and intent on their stylized poses and gestures. And not an iron bar in sight.

I confirmed Ramakrishna Alva's description of the cruel guru elsewhere, when my wife Feri and I visited Rukmini Devi Arundale in Madras. She is a noted teacher of classical dance-drama, whose husband was the Irishman G.S. Arundale, the author of *Kundalini, an Occult Experience* and of *Gods in the Becoming*. We met in the theosophy centre in Adyar, and when I mentioned Ramakrisha Alva's experience with his guru, she said:

'My teacher—most orthodox and old-fashioned—was a very severe taskmaster, and many dancers died young because of that. We were completely under the control of the teachers. I have tried to reform all that.'

But all of this notwithstanding, the willingess to revere saturates India. We found it in our travels across India, like the later experiences of Peter Brent. He faithfully reports this willingness in his book, warts, wonders, and all, as for example in the following:

Swami Akhanananda's devotees have produced a booklet, *Glimpses of Life Divine*, which gives details of his origins and development. The followers of most gurus bring out such pamphlets; sometimes even a biography, a full-fledged book. The story is always set out with great affection, eulogistically; no roughness is allowed to blur the hagiographic intent . . . The booklet tells of his devoted spiritual practice, of the addresses he has given and the people he has helped. It tells of the visions he has seen and the miracles he has performed. 'On one occasion a boy who had been dead for some time became an evil spirit and starting haunting and troubling his mother. No amount of treatment could cure the mother and ultimately the spirit of the dead boy spoke and requested recitation of Srimad Bhagwat [the *Bhagavad-Gita*] by a learned man. For this purpose a request was made to our Swamiji and he recited the Bhagwat Sapta and at the end the evil spirit declared that he had been freed from bondage and thereafter he never troubled or haunted anybody and his mother at once felt completely cured.[57]

Hagiography is the right word here, but in terms of living saints, not the safely dead and canonized kind. It is not a uniquely Hindu condition. In 1962 I visited Padre Pio, the stigmatist and 'living saint' of southern Italy. The abundance of healing (and other) miracles associated with this attractive and humble man embarrassed the Vatican, and when I was in his town, San Giovanni Rotondo, I saw a Lourdes Italian-style in the course of construction. Little plaques in the gift shops and on walls read, 'Padre Pio, pray for us', and pilgrims crowded to kiss his bandaged hand. Even the southern Communists praised the man with the wounds of Christ on his body while reviling the Church to which he belonged. There was a medievalism in the air and a sense of the numinous, just as I later found at certain shrines in India that were dedicated to a present or past giant of the spirit.

Whatever one feels about the devotionalism of the Hindus (or the southern Italians), however one may feel about the curious and powerful urge to adore living charismatics, one must accept the phenomenon of guruhood, and how it shades into avatarhood. Take, for example, the recent example of Barry Long in London, particularly as expressed in a quarter-page advertisement in *The Observer* of 17 February 1985.

'I am Guru,' runs the headline of the ad, 'Who are you?' Beside Long's head-and-shoulder picture there is an extensive text which is worth reproducing in its entirety but which I can only dip into here. The advertisement is a call for disciples that ends, 'Come when you can' to the Barry Long centre. It starts, however, with an intriguing binocular quality, as two Barry Longs speak to the reader with one voice:

Let me introduce myself. I am Barry Long, the person in this photograph. Now let me declare myself—for the person we say and think we are does not reveal who or what we are. And I do not want to mislead you. I am guru, the power behind the person and spiritual teacher Barry Long. There is only one guru—one divine or cosmic teacher—and I am that. Barry Long is one aspect of my teaching, one of my manifold lives. Since time began I have appeared consciously in the world, declaring myself through enlightened individuals. Enlightened individuals are those rare men, and even more rarely seen women, who have voluntarily given up—surrendered—their person, for my entry into their being as the truth of themselves.

There are echoes here of Krishna, the god who descends among men. There are also echoes of Buddha, the man who ascends beyond the gods. There also follows an almost standard declaration: the Teacher has now appeared, to be recognized by those 'who are ready to hear me and be with me'. This is the defensive clause in any contract with such a being: the messiah is protected from mass rejection, since those who reject him are by definition 'not ready' for him. The promises follow, the mystic come-on of 'you must be serious' and 'if you are ready for this fundamental change' and 'you are yearning for something you cannot name'. Barry Long, however, is guru, and he can name the nameless for you. He adds:

The word guru is from Sanskrit, the oldest and truest written language reflecting the truth of life on earth as it once was. When Sanskrit was an active language, guru, the truth, lived and spoke through many, many individuals, mostly the elders of the race. To grow old then was not to be geriatric . . . It was to mature into the dignity of being the living truth, the revered guide, the awakener . . . Westernised society has no word for guru nor concept of it, as it has no time for guru . . . Where is guru on earth today? Are you guru? Are your parents guru? Are your friends, teachers or leaders guru? . . .

My enlightenment of Barry Long allows me to perform the extraordinary work of publicly declaring myself to the Westernised world as I am doing now in this document . . . [As] this man Barry Long I speak to the Westernised mind not through the inevitable mystique of some dark-skinned guru from the East, but as a man of the West itself. Barry Long was born and has lived his life in the Westernised society. In all this I do not want you to get the impression that I am separate from Barry Long. There is no duality here, no person to come between and make a problem, a doubt. As the man I am fully responsible for what I say. I am quite able to confront the most intelligent minds and make sense of what I teach . . . Being myself I am extraordinarily simple. I am able to speak directly and simply to ordinary people who yearn for love and truth.

Barry Long is only one among an increasing number of Western claimants to guru-cum-avatar status. He can be compared, for example, with Da Free John in the United States, whose appeal is to rather sophisticated folk, not to 'ordinary people'. Da Free John's self-declaration is in the form of a complex book, *Nirvanasara: Radical Transcendentalism and the Introduction of Advaitayana Buddhism* (Dawn Horse Press, Clearlake, California, 1982), and makes a straightforward appeal to mystically-inclined intellectuals. The Indologist Georg Feuerstein has accepted Da Free John's claim, and in a foreword to *Nirvanasara* writes:

How does one introduce a great adept (*mahā-siddha*), a living Buddha, and his compassionate, prophetic teaching? In the following essay I have given my own answer to this question. I have tried to keep myself open to, and to faithfully represent, the teaching of Master Da Free John, while at the same time endeavoring to remain sensitive to the naturally skeptical posture which, I suspect, most readers will maintain while perusing this volume. I have written as one who has committed himself to a particular way of life, namely the spiritual path hewn out by Master Da. Simultaneously, I have brought to bear on my presentation whatever scholarly skills I have acquired in my professional career as an indologist . . . I consider myself most fortunate to have entered the ambience of one of the truly great spiritual Lights of today's world. Master Da Free John's compassionate presence has already greatly transformed my life. His Teaching has definitely lured me down from the fence on which I have been sitting uneasily for a good many years . . . I am aware that the stance I have taken in my introduction to this auspicious volume is incompatible with the current 'objective' fashion of science. But this has ceased to trouble me . . . I am grateful to have been given the opportunity to do *guru-seva* in the shape of this introduction, and I respectfully bow to Master Da Free John.

Shortly after the publication of *Nirvanasara*, Georg Feuerstein wrote to me in Canada, inviting me to consider Master Da's claim, later suggesting that I might wish to endorse it. I did not, but I felt a certain sympathy for Feuerstein in his move from neutral cultural anthropologist to respectful devotee. In my early twenties, I became a member of the Baha'i Faith, which meant that I accepted the claim of a Persian prophet, Baha'u'llah, to be 'the manifestation of God for this age'. His claim has had longer to establish and sanctify itself in a growing body of believers, but in objective terms it is a comparable claim to Da Free John's. I do not now see it as a unique modern revelation of truth, although I still admire the sweep and relevance of the Baha'i message. That relentless requirement to surrender one's psychological independence to The Other has long since eroded my own commitment to *any* transcendental claimant and impels me to ask what inspires the claim, what pushes people to start new movements, what causes their success and what causes—more frequently—their failure. It is, writ large, the same psychology as the Master and the Disciple.

One must go on asking these questions, precisely because 'guruitis' and messianism are so seductive. In Barry Long's declaration we see the guru-face of the phenomenon, while in Feuerstein's endorsement of Master Da we see the shishya-face, requiring the public immolation of one man's reputation as an 'objective' scholar. Whatever the compulsion to be received as a guru-avatar or to surrender to the charisma of such a claimant, the price exacted can be quite ferociously high. The private yet public contract between Master and Disciple must stand up to, and may in fact create, great strains. Bhagwan Shree Rajneesh's move from Poona to Oregon was attended at first by great expectations and some apparent results, but slid later, in 1985, into scandal and disintegration. Separately, in April of the same year, *The Observer* in London reported on Da Free John as follows: 'A tiny tropical isle in the Fijian chain, bought as a refuge for a California cult leader who calls himself Da Free John—a 5ft 9in, 16st, self-proclaimed incarnation of the deity—has become the scene of sex-and-drugs orgies, according to defectors from the sect. Former top-level aides of the "Master" . . . came forward last week with a stream of charges of brainwashing, faked miracles, physical abuse of women cultists and financial chicanery.'

And so on. Whether it is true almost does not matter; one can only be as cautious about this information as one is cautious about the introduction written by the convinced supporter. The kind of newspaper coverage instanced above is all too common in relation to gurus, Eastern or Western, who create ashram communes and seek utopian solutions to the world's problems, whether in Rishikesh in India or Rajneeshpuram in Oregon. By their fruits, I suppose, one comes to know them, as with all egregious figures in human history.

And yet, and yet . . . there *are* fruits. If not the ritualism of much of the *Vedas*, there is that fountain of inspired speculation, the *Upanishads*. Along with these often obscure but always provocative works there is the challenge of the *Gita* and the austere vigour of Patanjali. Excesses and orgies and rumours of excesses and orgies there have been in India and elsewhere down the years; authoritarianism and even acts of cruel domination have occurred and will occur; but none of them are ultimately the point. The venal and egoistical swamis co-occur with others whose faces reflect a most peculiar serenity. The system of yoga and Indian philosophy was created by *gurus* and has been sustained by *gurus* while at the same time it is clouded by *gurus* and brought into disrepute by *gurus*. Which makes it entirely and typically human. The ideal, however, cannot be tarnished—no matter how much karma cola is bottled and distributed.

I have no doubt that the claims will continue, and new *shishyas* will flock to new *gurus*. There may, however, develop other concepts of teacher and disciple that place less emphasis on absolute control on the one side and dazed devotion on the other. If so, it is just conceivable that this will help liberate both the teachers and the disciples from roles that are hard for mortal egos to sustain. It should after all be possible to teach without needing to be God, and to learn without becoming a slave.

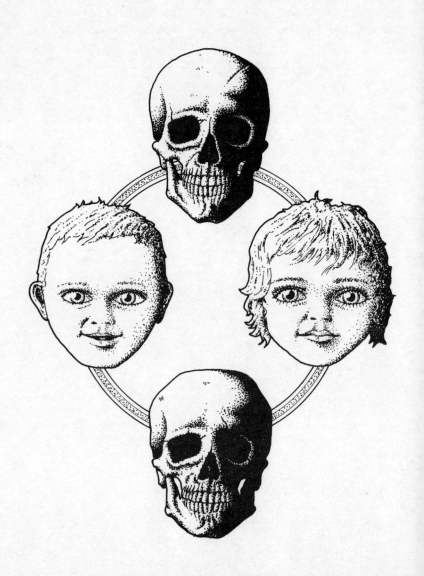

12. KARMA and SAMSARA

Pleasure is not the goal of man, but knowledge. Pleasure and happiness come to an end. It is a mistake to suppose that pleasure is the goal. The cause of all the miseries we have in the world is that men foolishly think pleasure to be the ideal to strive for. After a time man finds that it is not happiness, but knowledge, towards which he is going, and that both pleasure and pain are great teachers, and that he learns as much from evil as from good.

As pleasure and pain pass before his soul, they leave upon it different pictures, and the result of these combined impressions in what is called man's 'character'. If you take the character of any man, it really is but the aggregate of tendencies, the sum total of the bent of his mind; you will find that misery and happiness are equal factors in the formation of that character. Good and evil have an equal share in moulding character, and in some instances misery is a greater teacher than happiness. In studying the great characters the world has produced I dare say, in the vast majority of cases, it would be found that it was misery that taught more than happiness, it was poverty that taught more than wealth, it was blows that brought out their inner fire more than praise.

Like fire in a piece of flint, knowledge exists in the mind; suggestion is the friction that brings it out. So with all our feelings and actions—our tears and our smiles, our joys and our griefs, our weeping and our laughter, our curses and our blessings, our praises and our blames—every one of these we may find if we calmly study our own selves, to have been brought out from within ourselves by so many blows. The result is what we are. All these blows taken together are called Karma—work, action. Every mental and physical blow that is given to the soul, by which, as it were, fire is struck from it, and by which its own power and knowledge are discovered, is Karma, this word being used in its widest sense; thus we are all doing Karma all the time. I am talking to you: that is Karma. You are listening: that is Karma. We breathe: that is Karma. We walk: Karma. Everything we do, physical or mental, is Karma, and it leaves it marks upon us.[58]

Swami Vivekananda's is the classic Hindu view of *karma*, but not the only one. That view turns the simple everyday concept of 'doing' or 'action' into a cosmic principle that proposes the endless flow of cause into effect. This austere picture disdains such great Western ideals as 'life, liberty, and the pursuit of happiness', while at the same time piling action on effect and effect on action until we sag under the weight of the *karma* loaded upon us. This sense of a physical burden is not entirely unreasonable either, if we look at an older non-Hindu conception of what *karma* is and does.

Although the heretical sect of the Jains came into existence in the middle of the first millennium BC they claim to represent a truly ancient Indian tradition, and certainly their pessimistic conception of the universe is far more basic, austere, and uncompromising than that of the classical Hindus. Like Buddhism, Jainism crystallized in the area of what is now Bihar, brought to its peak by the ascetic sage Vardhamana. He was a contemporary of Gautama the Buddha's, and like him a prince who abandoned family life to become the saviour figure that his followers still call Mahavira, 'the Great Hero'. Mahavira saw himself not as the first spiritual conqueror or *jina*, but the last of a line of twenty-four stretching back to the dawn of time. Once, in the days of the first *jinas*, the human race had been gigantic and lived off the fruit of wishing trees. But over the aeons we have shrunk, and will go on shrinking till one day, at the very end of time, we will be dwarves in caves, without a single Jain left to explain reality to us. Then the vast impersonal cosmos will dissolve, and the whole inexorable cycle start again.

Jainism—ironically, the religion of the 'victors'—offers even less consolation than classical Hinduism and Buddhism: the world is truly a poor and painful place, where *jiva* ('spirit', 'living stuff') is bonded to *ajiva* ('matter', 'the unalive'). Spirit is in everything, in the rocks and trees as well as in animals and people, and longs for liberation. It can only, however, be liberated by the teachings of the *jinas*, which—if rigorously followed life after life—provide an eventual escape into an isolation (*kaivalya*) untainted by matter.

The Jains conceived the universe as a vast man, while the liberated soul is a kind of bubble of relief that rises to a lonely bliss at the top of the cosmic skull. This release can be achieved only in one way: by reversing the processes by which *jiva* and *ajiva* became entangled in the first place. In some mysterious way at the beginning of time, before the happy giants and their wishing trees existed, the atoms of spirit began to be covered in tiny flecks of non-spirit, stuff that stuck to them like dust on an oiled surface. Their naturally bright essences became obscured—the more dust, the greater obscurity—until we reached the condition in which we exist today. So much of this dust has fallen on us, speck by insidious speck, that we have acquired physical bodies in a physical world, and our spirits are completely hidden.

This clinging dust, in the Jain view, is *karma*. We are covered, embalmed, entombed in *karma*, and the more we act in the world the more the *karma* covers and binds us. That is the true horror of existence, as judged by the Jains. To lift this obscuring blight, the sole formula is not more action but less: to defeat *karma* one must cease to act, and if possible cease to accept our sheaths of flesh. The greatest and most meritorious Jain act is suicide through self-starvation. Mahavira himself set the example in this, and if we can follow that example then our karmic burden will certainly force us to be born again, but in a slightly finer state. Further lives of relentless inaction followed by suicide will slough off our burden layer by layer, until at last in some future demise we too can rise, like the twenty-four *jinas*, to float free in the upper reaches of the cosmic skull.

There is no god who can help us in this; the gods too are trapped. Only the *jinas* light the way, cool, blank-eyed saviours who exemplify, but do not lend a hand. In a grim universe, we are each alone in our struggle with the blight of *karma*.

In the tapestry of world-negation that India has been weaving for centuries, Jainism is the most negative pattern of them all. It is no surprise that the fortunes of this movement have waned, nor that the Jains expected them to wane, painting a picture of the universe in which their message would never really make much difference. Compared to them, the Buddhists are giddy optimists and the Hindus are hedonists in love with the wheel of birth and death.

Among the Hindus, *karma* is two-fold. Firstly, there is the impact that it has on our lives: psychic rather physical motes that settle on our divine mirrors and obscure their ability to reflect God. Additionally, however, there is *karma* as one's bounden duty, the kind of 'right' action that one must engage in, as a member of a certain caste, with a certain occupation, and specific obligations to one's ancestors, family, society and god(s). This *karma* pairs off with another vigorous concept, *dharma*, that represents the proper ordering of both universe and society, and of an individual life in that universe and that society. Right *dharma* prevents wrong *karma* from accumulating upon the sheaths of the spirit. More, it promotes right *karma*, and in the long term that kind of *karma* is a lot easier to get rid of than the other kind. In the end, however, all *karma*, bad and good, must go in the process of liberation—the heavy nasty stuff first, then the passionate forceful stuff, and finally the light spiritual stuff. Only when the last of it has gone can one step off the wheel.

The Hindu view of things differs from the Western view in various ways, not the least of which is the nature of time and action. In the West, at least in recent centuries, time has been conceived more or less as a straight line, running from the past through the present into the future. It is also conceived as a line that has dipped down from Eden and begun to ascend again since Christ. Additionally, it is conceived as an upward line by rationalists and evolutionists, up from the slime of ancient seas to modern humanity, the acme of biosocial achievement. The twentieth century is less sanguine about this view of things than were our nineteenth-century predecessors, but when we think about things like 'progress', 'growth', education' and the like we are still largely linear in the way we conceive and depict the passage of time.

The dials of our clocks, however, are round, and the sweep of hour, minute, and second hand all portray time as circles within circles. This is closer to the Eastern view, particularly to the Hindu conception of vast cycles of time (*kalpas*) within which there are lesser ages (*yugas*). These cyclic epochs move to the rhythm of lesser gods serving greater Gods who create, sustain, and then dissolve the world only to start the process again and again—and again.

In the West, we fear death and worry about whether there is anything beyond the grave. In India they fear both death and the repetition of death, life and the repetition of life. It is hard to tell whether this is a larger fear, or just the same fear expressed in a different way, but certainly it has been powerful enough to transcend ancient Vedic beliefs in heavens and hells that were rather like recent Western beliefs. Hindus still believe in paradises and purgatories, but these are just *other* lives—super-lives or sub-lives, but still less than the proper goal. Even the gods take shape and dissolve. Everything does that, from the lowest to the highest. The wheel of *samsara* is vast beyond conception, and everything in existence is bound to it, bound to repeat in slightly varied forms all the potentialities of the wheel. From a God's-eye view, being born as a flea or a prince or a god called Indra is much the same, just variations on a common theme.

The majority view in India is still that the wheel is onerous, but not everyone believes this. Many Tantric saints and sinners have found the wheel of *samsara*, which is *maya* in a different form, as intriguing and as worthwhile as the void beyond it. 'Who seeks nirvana?' asks the Tantric saint with a grin. If you seek it, seek it here and now, not there and then. For such an adept, the wonders of the sensory world are to be savoured and used—*bhoga* or worldly satisfaction is a necessary complement to *yoga* or otherworldly effort.[59] Not all Tantrics have agreed about the

worth of body, woman, and world, but the strongest view in India is still
the vision of the renunciant, although here and there and now and again
one can celebrate *samsara*.

Samsara is the running round of the wheel, all the twining threads of
maya, everything that flows, that changes, that cannot stay long in one
knot or shape. Fresh whirls and eddies appear—you and me; fresh knots
are tied and loosened—me and you. Something of us, however, passes
from embodiment to embodiment, as if a kind of long-drawn-out
process of education were at work. The basic Indian theories of
metempsychosis, the transmigration of souls, are each logical within
their own Hindu, Buddhist, or Jain frameworks. Each proposes a vast
and intricate universe of relationships, and each also proposes certain
shortcuts through the maze of lives and deaths. The promise that each
system makes to its adherents is that, if they wish, they can short-circuit
samsara and *maya*.

Hence the teachings of sages like Yajnavalkya, Kapila, Gautama the
Buddha, Vardhamana called Mahavira, Patanjali, and the existence of
the *Upanishads*, the *Gita*, the *Hathayoga-Pradipika*, and so on. All the
yogas or techniques and *margas* or paths are aimed at transcending
samsara, and at providing certain embodied powers and benefits along
the way. They are all tough-minded, all agree about the need for
commitment, and all treat *karma* and the *samskaras* as the first issues to
be overcome.

One has to be careful here, because the word *samskara* looks so much
like the word *samsara*. The prefix *sa-*, *sam-*, or *san-* (often nasalized),
appears in such words as 'samadhi', 'samyama', 'samsara', 'samskara',
'Sankhya', and 'Sanskrit' itself. It is a distant cousin of the *co-* or *com-*
(etc.) in words of Latin origin like 'co-worker', 'communicate',
'connect', 'colleague', 'cognition', etc. It means 'with', 'together',
'completely', and may suggest something shared or united. *Samadhi* is
therefore 'putting or getting everything together' (integration);
samyama is a reining in of one's powers, concentrating them all in one;
samsara is everything running around together—while the *samskaras* are
from the same root as *karma* (*kri*, 'to do, to act'), and are all the actions
and results of actions in all existence and all lives. Massed *karma*, in
effect.

The theory is broadly agreed across the spectrum of Hindu thought.
Each of us exists as sheaths within sheaths, a multiple being and not an
indivisible individual. Our grosser physical sheaths are (at least
symbolically) on the outside, and the progressively subtler (but still
physical) sheaths come one within the other like boxes in a Chinese
puzzle. At the core of the sheaths (at least symbolically) is something

which is not a sheath but sheathed, like a sword. It is not physical. Some call it the *jiva* ('living one'), others the *atma* or *atman* ('soul' or 'self'), and others again combine the two as the *jivatma(n)* ('the living soul'). For some the living soul is in an ultimate sense the same stuff as the sheaths that shield it or obscure it; for others it is a brighter and better thing altogether, and beyond description. For all, however, the *samskaras* or general burden of *karma* stand between it and ourselves becoming properly aware of it—and between it and its proper state of freedom.

The school called *Vedanta* has a well-delineated model of sheaths and sheathed, in which one *jivatman* relates to three *shariras* ('bodies') associated with five *koshas* ('sheaths'). In tabular form, the bodies and sheaths are as follows:

shariras ('bodies')	*koshas* ('sheaths')
1. *sthula-sharira* (the gross body)	1. *annamaya-kosha* (the food-creating sheath)
2. *sukshma-sharira* (the subtle body)	2. *pranamaya-kosha* (the breath/life-creating sheath)
	3. *manomaya-kosha* (the mind-creating sheath)
	4. *vijnanamaya-kosha* (the knowledge-creating sheath)
3. *karana-sharira* (the causal body)	5. *anandamaya-kosha* (the bliss-creating sheath)

This double system is, like any other theoretical or descriptive system, a set of intellectual categories invented by human beings, although some will argue that they were revealed as ultimate truth by gods or inspired sages. There is no valid reason, however, for seeing them as other than constructs like a model of the atom or a map of the North Atlantic. They do seek, however, to catch in a classifier's net something of reality, and express a belief in a hierarchy of elements in each of us, shading from the heavy and material up and up to the infinitely bright and light and refined. As such, this is itself a refinement of the Jain theory of *jiva* trapped in *ajiva*. It is broadly speaking an analogue of the Western idea of a basic body ruled by a subtler mind serving an eternal spirit. Like many Westerners, however, who do not see the body/mind/spirit picture as a theory at all, many thoughtful Hindus do not see the body-and-sheath model as a 'theory'. It is simply the tradition that they are used to, and the one that has helped them for centuries to think about life and death.

In addition, this hierarchy of human parts has the same ladder-like quality as the Buddha's Eight-Fold Path and Patanjali's Eight-Limb Yoga. As you consider it, you are forced to climb mentally from the lowest to the highest, a vertical scale that is common in the cultural and intellectual traditions of India and ranges from the structures of the caste system to the four-fold structure of the life-plan of caste Hindu men, the four *ashramas*. We appear to be dealing here with an archetypal aspect of Indian thought and action.

Western occultists have tended to tie in this Eastern vision of bodies, sheaths, and spirit with their own conception of planes or levels of existence: physical, astral, and etheric bodies all serving the spirit. The parallelism is striking. It suggests, as the occultist argues, that down the centuries there has been an esoteric doctrine available to the gnostic few: 'secret teachings' about life and death that have come down from ancient sources. It is a belief worth careful assessment. Migrant groups, from the Mongols to the Gypsies, have moved from East to West; Indian numbers became our 'Arabic' numbers and are used everywhere today, including the magic symbol zero without which mathematicians would be at a loss. It is quite possible that from one or more sources a common coherent body of beliefs has disseminated around the world and is sustained by groups of like-minded people, who initiated their successors into their various lodges. Alchemists, Rosicrucians, Freemasons, and others demonstrate at least a gnostic mentality if not the existence of unbroken lines of Those Who Know, a hidden priesthood of the truly well informed guarding a precious heritage, or at least sharing a certain kind of sociocultural unity.

I am, however, wary of conspiracy theories, even conspiracies of white magicians and wise adepts. It seems far more likely that the various theories of body, mind, and spirit have grown up in overlapping cultural situations, acting and interacting as sharp minds met each other in various places and at various times. In this way Pythagoras could be a Western analogue of Kapila, while the Neoplatonists of Europe could have something in common with Tantrics in Hinduism and Buddhism. There also appears to be a genuine unity of mystical experience: human beings seeking a 'higher' awareness appear everywhere to have reported the same phenomena, whatever symbolism they may have used. In that way, it should be no surprise that Zen might have echoes among the Sufis, and yogic practices resemble the hesychasm of Greek Orthodox monks.

It is therefore easy enough to align the Indian theory of bodies, sheaths, and spirit with Western occult ideas of various planes and with the general religious tradition of body, mind, and spirit; but it is not so easy to align it with current Western scientific thinking. Unlike the other belief systems. Western science is essentially materialist. Traditional religions are dualistic, placing matter on one side and spirit on the other. Occultists and Indian philosophers are more flexible, in that they grade the physical, shading it delicately towards the spirit. Western science, even when practised by religious people, is by definition matter-based, and either will never 'discover' spirit because spirit doesn't exist, or has not yet found any way of coming to terms with spirit. Indeed, it is still struggling to come to terms with *mind*.

Yet there is a certain reassuring strength to the Vedantist model when it is looked at 'scientifically'. In broad terms, the first Hindu body is the one we can touch and feel, the one that moves around. The second is its mental partner, the motor that runs it, while the third is evidently our karmic experience, a response to all the environments and activities we have ever known. Separately, the five sheaths are firstly our anatomy of blood, bone, and flesh, then secondly a kind of breath-related physiology, then a neurological analogue, then the upper centres of the brain, and fifthly the 'superconsciousness' of which those brain centres often give us clues. That would be *buddhi*, the higher intellect and focus of enlightenment.

So some kind of fitting together is possible, but no easier for the body-and-sheath picture than for the *chakras* and *kundalini*. No neat fit is ever possible between such different systems of thought, but it may well be possible to use the Western and Eastern theories as components in a fuller theory of human nature that can integrate both, as well as drawing in, say, Chinese Taoist and Japanese Zen thinking.

The crucial issue here, however, is the relationship between the various levels of 'bodiness' and that Other which is said to incarnate ('become en-fleshed'). But what exactly moves on after death? As regards this conundrum, A.L. Basham is particularly clear and concise:

The belief in karma does not necessarily involve fatalism. A fatalist strain often appears in Hindu thought, but most teachers disapproved of it. Our present condition is inevitable, but only because of the karma accruing from our past deeds. We cannot escape the law of karma any more than we can escape the law of gravity or the passage of time, but by judgement and forethought we can utilize the law of karma to our own advantage.

The process of transmigration was interpreted somewhat variously, but all schools agreed that the soul does not transmigrate in a state of nudity, but with a sheath or series of sheaths of subtle matter; the condition of the sheaths depends on the balance of previous good and evil karma, and the new birth is determined by the nature of the sheaths around the soul. The subtle body of transmigration is deprived of sense organs, including mind, the sixth sense, and therefore the soul cannot normally remember previous births or the passage from one body to another. Very advanced souls, however, can sometimes recapture memories of previous existences, and some sects evolved a special technique for doing so.[60]

Remembering past lives . . . That is an area of discussion fraught with problems, although some hardy scientific investigators have begun to make tentative studies of people who claim to remember such lives. Patanjali specifically indicates that at an advanced stage on the yogic journey an adept will begin to recall past-life experiences. If something like that happens—and it appears to be the case that *something* quite startling can happen to yogis and others—then it falls into one of three categories, depending on what you can persuade yourself to believe: it is an imaginative fiction, a hallucinatory experience of great scientific interest, but not more than that; it is possession by a well-informed or imaginative entity, an invader of one's personality, perhaps the kind of devil that Jesus cast out; or it *is* the resurfacing of deep memory, which means not only that there is a transmigratory 'essence' but also that memory does not depend on the physical world in order to keep its shape. All it needs, like music broadcast through the air, is a machine to transform it back into a hearable form.

In India I found it easy to live and think in terms of reincarnation. It was in the cultural air all around. The Judaeo-Christian-Islamic-Baha'i line of religions, however, does not give any credit whatever to the transmigration of souls, although individuals and groups within that tradition have been and are sometimes surprisingly well disposed towards the idea of multiple lives in this world. Reincarnation is certainly no more or less reasonable than any other set of beliefs about life and life after death. Science, however, resists metaphysical and mystical views of life, and currently (and for the foreseeable future) will have little to say about either a single super-life after death or a string of lives past and lives to come. There is no evidence acceptable to physicists, chemists, biologists, psychologists, and anthropologists that metempsychosis fuels the processes of life in this world of ours.

To believe in reincarnation is therefore to venture beyond the bounds of Western scientific rationalism as presently laid out. To an occultist, that is not of course a drawback; it is a basic tenet of the various occult movements that Western science is still only toying with the nature of reality. For people who are conventionally religious, however, there is either no problem or a large problem. If you are a Hindu, a Jain, or a Buddhist, reincarnation is so basic and believable that there is no need to discuss it; it is taken for granted in the same way that one takes air or clothes or Monday for granted. But if you are a sincere and fairly orthodox Jew, Christian, Muslim, or Baha'i, you are not supposed to entertain reincarnation as a basic belief or as an option. It is out of the discussion in such worldviews. It is, in crude terms, heretical.

The situation is complicated, however, by the fact that nowadays more and more people are less and less conventional in their sense of being religious. For everyone who takes refuge in the unyielding dogmas of a religion, there is someone else who wants freedom of speculation. A certain polarizing seems to be occurring here, between a retreat to fundamentalism and an edging out towards religious worldviews tailored to the individual. Both extremes have their risks. For those, however, who see themselves as Jews and Christians, etc., but not as always accepting the official line, reincarnation occupies a special shadow area. It has become an option, which may or may not be taken up, or which may be taken up on occasion, or which may be adopted as an *ad hoc* solution. In the last instance, it may be seen as a more bearable alternative to long ages in heaven, hell, purgatory, limbo, or some other permanent future non-physical address.

This, I suspect, is currently the position of many Westerners who are intrigued by and practise yoga in some degree. Aware that *karma* and *samsara* are keystones of the yoga arch, they feel constrained to give reincarnation some freedom of movement in their minds. If they are serious about the subject, they would seem to have little alternative.

13. MANTRA and YANTRA

With respect to every *mantra*—as in the case of Western ceremonial—there must be *intent*, otherwise the words of a parrot or of a gramophone would carry the full power. When magical incantations are used, and there are blessings meant to help or curses meant to injure, we must consider them in two classes—those recited in the presence of the person to be affected, and those recited apart from him, and even secretly.[61]

These are the words, not of a magician, but of Ernest Wood, in his classic book entitled simply *Yoga*. It was published by Penguin in 1959, and there have been one revision and many reprints since. Born in Manchester in 1883, Wood studied physics, chemistry, and geology, became an educational administrator in India, studied Sanskrit, Vedanta, and yoga, met Indian scholars and swamis, and wrote a variety of books on education, psychology, and Indian philosophy. Towards the end of a long life he was also president of the American Academy of Asian Studies, a graduate school in San Francisco.

He was a man who bridged both West and East. If he meant 'magic' he said magic, and if he meant 'science' he said science, as for example in this excerpt, from the introduction to *Yoga*:

There were in the old days in India strata of society which provided for men and families dedicated to religion and philosophy, and thus able to study and practise these without such distractions as we have in modern living. These groups gave themselves to this study in a definitely scientific and factual manner, with application in practice and pragmatic consideration of results. Yoga thus grew up as applied religion, and at the same time the science of introspectional psychology—introspectional meaning not retreat from factual experience, but direct inspection of the contents of the mind, yet not ignoring the application of the knowledge so gained to the body and the environment.[62]

In order to describe yoga, Wood wrote a book which seeks to synthesize East with West and science with the occult. He appears to have deliberately chosen to talk about certain Hindu traditions as

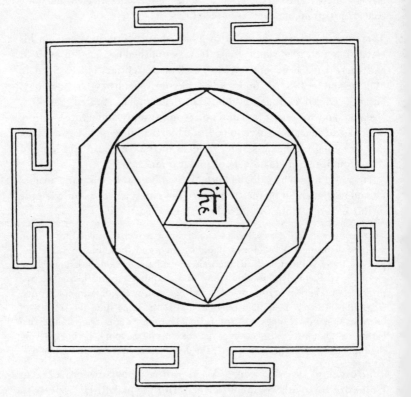

The Yantra of Liberation

'science' and as 'psychology' in order to push Westerners into putting them on a par with scientific disciplines born in Europe. This is a position that I sympathize with, but the angle of vision in 1986 is rather different from 1959. Today, it is no longer necessary to call Eastern disciplines by Western names in order to make them respectable. Nowadays it is important to see them as themselves, in their own settings, and not trick them out in borrowed clothes.

Yoga is not a science in any Western sense, nor a form of the Western mental analysis called 'psychology'. It can be investigated scientifically—and should be. It is psychologically interesting, certainly. But in principle it is as possible to look at science yogically as to look at yoga scientifically, and just as informative.

As a pioneer synthesizer of yoga, science, magic, and the occult, Wood could hardly be expected to create a seamless robe of a book. The stitching shows, as it shows in all such present-day works because they do not yet have an overview that contains both yoga and science, both science and magic, both science and the occult. We are a long way from that overview, and nothing demonstrates this more than a discussion of *mantra* and *yantra*. Wood is a fairly typical interpreter of such ideas, as for example when he observes that *mantras* said in the presence of a human target will have a 'musical effect' as well as a 'telepathic effect'. He notes that 'it is well known that different kinds of music excite or depress different parts and functions of the body', then goes on to assert that 'every word uttered in our hearing thus has some effect upon our minds and bodies'. For him the *mantra* is a focusing device as well as a sonic tool, focusing the mind of the transmitter and creating an effect on the mind and body of the target person or group. Wood also does not shrink from pointing out that *mantras* operate in the same domain as talismans and amulets: 'In this case, certain objects have had blessings or curses pronounced over them, and even willed into them, as it were.'[63]

There is no science as such in this, however, although Wood seeks a working relationship between science on one side and various matters which would nowadays he called 'paranormal' on the other. Telepathy is not part of established psychology. Many people believe in it, or would like to believe in it, or are fascinated by the possibility of thought transmission, but science does not currently endorse its existence. Thought transmission, however, is important to Wood and to many others in their discussion of *mantra*, as he makes abundantly clear in the following statement:

To understand this feature of what to the layman appears to be a piece of magic, one must take into account that thoughts not only travel from one mind to another—like letters through the post—and impress the mind of the receiver according to his sensitiveness, but actually impress or cling to objects.

This is an interesting supposition, but that is all it is in terms of scientific inquiry. Wood goes on to describe in general terms 'some experiments which I conducted over fifty years ago', where sets of blank cards of an unspecified kind were 'impressed' by means of concentrated thought with pictures of various common objects. After shuffling, a 'sensitive' blindfolded subject then described the 'thought picture' which had been impressed on various cards, 'and in this case was right every time'. Wood then says: 'For this reason almost all people get some impressions of thought and feeling (emotion) from the objects they handle. Thus a book which has been well read will convey more than one new from the press.'[64]

Which may all be true, but we do not objectively know that it is so. Occultism may accept the propositions that Wood is putting forward here; indeed, as occult arguments they are entirely legitimate. In the garb of science, however, they are misleading. Wood's remarks here are not scientific at all, because we have no access to the findings of that experiment conducted fifty years earlier, we do not know the conditions under which it was conducted, and we have no means of replicating it. The statements have no statistical worth, and belong in some kind of pre-scientific limbo. They have in fact to be taken on trust, which makes them essentially religious statements. And most disturbing of all, the statement 'what to the laymen appears to be a piece of magic' suggests a state of grace possessed by the writer (and some unknown others) which excludes the 'lay' person (apparently the bulk of the readers).

However, the lay person would actually be right, as Wood was right at the start. We enter the landscape of magic when we talk about *mantras*.

In Sanskrit a *mantra* can be many related things. At root, it is a thought (*man*) device (*tra*). In Hindu society at large it was and is a form of prayer and can also be a hymn, a sacred text, a mystical verse, a magic spell, and a secret design. In tandem, a *yantra* is at root a restraining (*yan*) device (*tra*), a means of holding in, concentrating or focusing the mind-cum-will. With *yantras*, however, this is usually done through the eyes or visualization, while with *mantras* one operates through the vocal cords. And if that makes you think of magicians pronouncing incantations while drawing circles and triangles on the floor, then you are being entirely reasonable, because that is what is going on. In combination in Sanskrit, a *mantra-yantra* is an amulet with a magic formula on it, and in present-day Hindi *jantar-mantar* has much the same connotation as both magic and 'mumbo-jumbo' in English—what street magicians say and do during their conjuring tricks.

One way of viewing such devices of sound, thought, and shape is to do what Wood clearly did—accept an ancient magical side to yoga that is still powerful in India today. As with *asanas*, one can then say that useful 'real' therapeutic practices have emerged out of this ancient background just as chemistry emerged out of alchemy and astronomy emerged out of astrology. If some people once searched for the philosopher's stone, to turn base metals into gold, we are all the beneficiaries, because today we have the wonders of the chemist's art and science.

That is a legitimate response. But there is an additional dimension that we cannot ignore, and that many of the people who are interested in yoga have no intention of ignoring. That is the magical realm in its own right—not as something which the human race has outgrown, or ought by now to have outgrown, or that education will help us outgrow shortly, but something which is built into us, that has been with us far longer than rationalism, science, and education in the modern sense. 'Magic' here is a certain way of appreciating (and manipulating) the world and ourselves. No modern rational development has in fact banished this aspect of humanity, and calling it 'voodoo' or 'superstition' in order to banish it is itself an appeal to the power of magic. This is not to argue that magic is 'right' or 'desirable', or 'better' than science or anything else; it is a question of recognizing a stratum of thought and behaviour that will not and probably cannot go away. People will buy amulets, use love potions, consult oracles, read omens, check their star charts, bless and curse much as they have done for uncounted ages, whether they can account for what they are doing or not, and whether they are proud of what they are doing or not. It is the oldest form of insurance in the world, and it has its own logic and momentum. Fingers crossed and touch wood.

Yoga taps, and has always tapped, into this stratum of thought and behaviour, and it is not the only system that does so. Faith healing does it obviously, where a physician's bedside manner and placebos do so more indirectly. Voodoo rites do it obviously, whereas a Christian priest's blessings and prayers do so more indirectly. Medicine men have always believed in interpreting dreams as magical guidance; scientists who find solutions to their problems in a dream have simply dreamt the solution—but the dream does its work regardless of our attitudes to it. For good or for ill, right or wrong, astronomy has never made astrology go away, and more people appear to be interested in what the stars 'say' than in what astronomers say about the stars. (It is probably—incidentally—as easy and useful to believe in sun signs, the Zodiac, and planetary aspects as it is to believe in black holes, light years, space-time continuums, cosmic rays and the Big Bang theory.)

Human beings everywhere appear at some time or other to have believed that the world is alive with spirits and potencies, and that people with magical power could pass it on, make it work, and change the world by means of either or both controlled utterances and special shapes and diagrams. This is as true of chanting among the Sioux and the sand paintings of the Navajo as it is true of chanting among the Hindus and their geometric *yantras*. Western science sits uneasily on top of this mass of ancient and persistent belief and behaviour—and sometimes looks suspiciously like magic and religion itself, as it pronounces its own mantras and draws its own yantras. My own suspicion is that there is a single continuum of human experience that unites magic, religion, and science—and unites them with yoga. Curiosity, fear, and a desire for power and security would appear to lie at the root of all such phenomena.

Georg Feuerstein describes *mantras*, *yantras* and the like as 'triggers' of a psychological nature: 'There is no single equivalent for *mantra* in any of the European languages, and the usual translation with "sacred syllable" is only an emergency equation. A *mantra* may be defined as a . . . series of phonemes [individual elements of sound] arranged according to conventional patterns in esoteric schools and, what is more important, transmitted from teacher to disciple in a more or less formal initiation. Thus the famous syllable *om*, representing the Absolute according to hindu [*sic*] tradition, on its own cannot be said to be a *mantra*; it becomes a *mantra* only when it is given by a teacher. A *mantra* is sound charged with numinous power.'[65] A loaded sound, like the 'loaded' bone that Australian aboriginal witch-doctors would point at the accused or accursed, causing them to die, or like the pins placed in voodoo dolls.

Ernest Wood agrees: '*Mantras* cannot be made by everybody. They have to be provided through or by a competent seer (*mantrakara*). In the case of Om, the source of it is regarded as nothing less than the triple divinity; it came to man as a revelation, not as a construct of his own.'[66]

Hindu teachers say less about the theory and practice of *mantras* than do Western observers, probably because their efficacy is taken for granted. Your guru gives you your *mantra* to be used by you and you alone, and you say it as specified, so many times a day as a kind of spiritual medicine. The assumption is that, if you repeat it as part of your *sadhana* or spiritual discipline regularly enough—in the technique known as *mantra-yoga* or in the repetitive process called *japa*—then you will one day cease to need to use it consciously. It will be established in you as a permanent focusing device—and will go on endlessly saying itself.

The *mantras* or 'thought forms', as Alain Daniélou calls them, are conceived as subtle entities in their own right and fuse with the subtle levels of our personalities. They are part of the belief that Sanskrit is a perfect magical vehicle. The *mantras*, like the language itself, have to be kept as free from corruption as possible—whence presumably the idea of their being passed with care and special power from guru to shishya. Complex *mantras* like the Buddhist *Om mani padme hum* ('Lo, the jewel is in the lotus') are basic prayer-frames, differing little from the Catholic Christian *Nomine Patris, et Filii, et Spiritus Sancti* ('In the Name of the Father, the Son, and the Holy Ghost/Spirit'). They are important, but more important and basic than these are the *bija-mantras* ('seed thought-forms').

A *seed mantra* is a single syllable like *OM/AUM*. It expresses an essential pre-linguistic fact, quality, thought, action, hope or whatever. The following is a selection of such primal syllables:

AIM for knowledge and fluency
HRIM for conquest over nature and an understanding of *maya*
KRIM for losing one's fear of death and gaining immortality
GLAUM for great mental powers
STRAUM to create lust
KHA for killing

OM or *AUM*, however, is the prince of *mantras*, and in the *Mandukya Upanishad* has a treatise to itself—short but significant among the classical *Upanishads*. The four *Vedas*, which are the scriptural foundation of orthodox Hinduism, are traditionally said to be no more than commentaries on this one syllable, which starts at the back of the mouth, travels over the tongue and closes with the lips in a long final nasal resonance. The first element, the vowel *A*, symbolizes the waking state in the microcosm of the individual and the state of creation in the macrocosm of the universe. The second element, the vowel *U*, is the dream state in an individual and the time of existence and manifestation in the universe (when God dreams the dream of *maya*). The third element, the nasal *M*, is the deep, dreamless state in you and me, and is dissolution in the cosmos, before the process starts again. The repetition of *AUM* is the cyclic condition of life, of breathing, of the coming and going of the ages.

But beyond the three conjoined sounds is a fourth element, *turiya*. It is the silence after the last resonance and before the process starts again.

It is the abiding stillness of transcendence and release. In terms of yoga breathing, *A* is the in-drawn breath, *U* is the retained breath, *M* is the exhaled breath, and *turiya* is the period of emptiness in the lungs before the next breath is taken in. In terms of the great god-figures, *A* is Brahma the Creator, *U* is Vishnu the Preserver, and *M* is Shiva or Shankara, the Destroyer/Dissolver, while *turiya* is the ultimate underlying all three, by whatever names that ultimate may be known in any particular sect. It is no surprise, therefore, that the *Mandukya Upanishad* says: 'This syllable Aum is the whole of existence.'

Where a *mantra* is thought as sound, a *yantra* is thought as a formal diagram. Thought can also be framed in other ways in Hinduism, as for example by a physical *asana*, a gesture or *mudra*, or through an image or 'idol', a *murti*. These various ways of enshrining thought can also co-occur, as for example when the statue of a god makes gestures, adopts a special pose, and is associated with written symbols and geometric designs. Hinduism is seldom miserly with its symbols: The more you have, the surer the focus and the effect. Insurance, again.

Much as *mantras* are based upon certain primal syllables, *yantras* are built up out of a variety of primary or stylized components, such as points, lines, triangles, squares, swastikas, lotuses, and circles. They all have mystical-cum-numerological values, and together make up the various yantric symbol-clusters that can be read by those who know the code.

Thus, a single point or *bindu* represents the place where world and spirit meet—the infinitesimal moment-place where manifestation starts. Once manifestation has occurred, it can 'travel' in one direction and be shown as a single line, or in four directions at right angles to each other, and be shown as a cross. When lines join up as triangles, they may point upwards or downwards. If upwards, they are phallic and fiery, and represent the masculine force known as Shiva. If downwards, they are vaginal or uterine and watery, and represent the feminine force of Shakti. If touching tip to tip, they make up Shiva's drum, an hourglass shape that represents dissolution. If entwined as a Star of David shape, they are god and goddess embraced, and represent the world as it is, created and on-going. When the embracing triangles split up into innumerable miniatures of themselves, they represent the universe of forms and interactions—the many created out of the two who are ultimately one (and a symbolic pattern that India shares with the Taoists of China).

Particularly intriguing to read is the *Mukti-yantra*, the Diagram of Liberation. In its centre sits the mantric syllable *HRIM*, the *bija-maya* or Seed of Illusion. Around it is a small square, which is earth, around that the fire triangle that is in turn inside the water triangle that is inside the hexagonal symbol of air that is embedded in the circle or wheel of existence, all in turn inside an octagon for the eight directions and the four-gated city of the world itself. These represent all the elements of the phenomenal world that the spiritual aspirant must understand and 'see through' on the way to *mukti* or final release from *maya*.

Where linear, flowing sound provides focus and power through the voice, the two-dimensional spread of a yantric diagram creates a visible frame for the student's thoughts. It shapes or constrains those thoughts, channelling them in the right direction. The concrete image can be drawn into the mind's eye, or the structure can be assembled imaginatively without such a physical diagram being present. This kind of visualization is important in many forms of yoga, but particularly so in Tantra, and significant when it comes to imagining the nature and power of the *chakras* or centres of energy in the body. Each chakra is, in fact, conceived as a yantric form.

Georg Feuerstein sees a *yantra* as 'a cosmogram or psychocosmogram —a codified map of the primary structure of phenomenal reality. It recaptures in simple geometrical form the process of the emergence of the Many from the One. The basic components of the *yantra* are the triangle, either upwards pointing (as *śiva*) or downwards pointing (as *śakti*), the circle, lotus petals, and the square and the point symbolizing the world axis':

The *yantra* may be drawn on paper, wood, cloth or any other material or *ex tempore* into sand. Also three-dimensional models are known. In the higher stages of tantric yoga, the *yantra* must be internalized, that is the *yogin* must build up the complex geometrical pattern mentally through the process of visualization. The *yantra* is erected either from the innermost point, called *bindu*, outwards—in accordance with the process of macrocosmic evolution— or from the outermost circumference towards the centre—in alignment with the microcosmic process of meditative involution.

After having established the *yantra* internally, the *yogin* next proceeds to dissolve it again without losing the heightened intensity of awareness which he has acquired during the visualization process. Since the *yogin* is, in consciousness, identical with the structure of the *yantra*, its dissolution necessarily implies his own extinction as an experiencing subject. If successful, the gradual demolition of the *yantra* catapults him into pure Being where all subject and object distinctions are invalid.[67]

As with all the psychic and physical techniques of yoga and other related Indian systems, the goal never varies. *Mantra, yantra, mudra, asana* and other aids—taken together or separately, one of them in the foreground or all of them given equal status—are no more and no less than props or stations along the inner way. The goal is always the same: seeing the one behind the many, transcending the opposites or dualities, surfacing out of *maya* into awareness. The goal in fact is *turiya*, the fourth condition, which lies beyond every *mantra* or *yantra* that was ever conceived.

14. MAYA and LILA

One day the god Vishnu appeared to the sage Narada.

'Your austerity and your devotion have been great,' he said. 'I therefore grant you a boon.'

Narada gazed in wonder at his visitor, and finally summoned up enough courage to say: 'Lord, explain your *maya* to me—explain that wonderful magic power.'

'Certainly,' said the god, 'if that is what you want.' He smiled a sublime, ambiguous smile, and said: 'Come with me.'

From the pleasant shade of the hermit's grove Vishnu led his disciple out into the open light of day. The sun blazed down, and as they walked farther and farther, without any mention of boons or *maya*, both became more and more thirsty. Finally, Vishnu sat down in the shade of a cliff and asked Narada to get him some water from a pool that lay some distance away.

'Of course, Lord,' said the hermit, and went to the pool. But when he bent over the pool to fill a pitcher with water he felt dizzy and fell in. When he managed to get out again, things seemed subtly different, and he found that a beautiful young woman had also come to fill a pitcher at the pool. She greeted him modestly, and invited him as a weary traveller to come and rest in her father's house. Seduced by her wonderful, ambiguous eyes, Narada followed her, forgetful of all else—indeed, unable to remember anything else.

He went with the girl, met her father, stayed with them day after day, and in due course began to work for the father, and with the passage of the months became like a son to him. In due course he married the young woman, and for twelve happy years lived with her, inheriting the patch of land and raising a family of three.

But there came a year of terrible floods, and in the awful wind and rain their hut was destroyed. In seeking high ground for safety, Narada one by one lost his beloved children and finally his dear wife was ripped

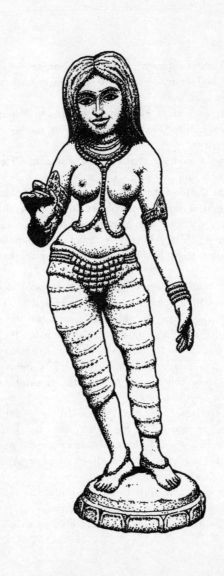

from his side. He himself was swept away on the torrent and, half-conscious, was eventually stranded on a stony beach. When he came to himself, all he could see was a plain of mud, and all he could do was weep. But as he wept, he heard a voice saying, as if from a great distance:

'Child, child, where is the water? I have been waiting for quite some time.'

And there was no mud and ruin, but only the hot sun overhead and Vishnu with his gentle, unyielding ambiguous smile.

There are many versions of this story. Sri Ramakrishna, the nineteenth-century Bengali saint, told one like it, and also had a tale to show that, whatever ultimate reality might be, it lies beyond our conventions of good and evil, fortune and misfortune—just as Narada discovered. He would tell of a personal vision that came one day when he was meditating on the steps of a sacred *tank* or pool. He also saw a beautiful woman coming towards him, and as he watched he saw that she was pregnant. Her belly swelled as he gazed at her, and she gave birth—there, on the steps—to a child of great beauty. Lovingly she cradled the babe, but as she caressed it she began to change once more. This time, however, she turned into a terrible, ravening creature which devoured the child before his eyes.

That woman, said Ramakrishna, was Time herself, Mother Kali, which produces everything and destroys everything with equal impartiality. Ultimate reality lies beyond both a mother's tender love and the worst excesses of monsters, all of which are bound up in the infinite web of *maya*.

Maya in Sanskrit is marvellous creative power—an art, a device, a trick, even fraud and jugglery. It can be witchcraft, an illusion, or a phantom, but above all else it is, particularly as described in the Vedanta school, the power which causes one to suppose that this world of which we are so apparently concrete a part is the truly real. Compared to higher reality, however, all of this world is illusion, a phantasmagoria that is sometimes pleasant, sometimes painful, and always transient and changing.

Maya is always presented as female, which may explain why so many sects and schools of yoga have recoiled from women. Or it may have been the other way round, that because women were so fatefully attractive, men with an urge for ascetic self-control saw them as snares. Monasticism around the world has often depicted women in this way, and even while rejecting individual earthly wives have transferred their enthusiasms to some kind of celestial woman, whether it is Ramakrishna's Kali the Mother, or the Virgin Mary adored by the monks of Athos in Greece, or the Shakti of Tantrism, the Tara of Tantric Buddhism, or Isis, Cybele, and many other goddess figures who have made stern demands on men. Even the *kundalini* serpent in Tantra and hatha-yoga is female—and to be preferred.

The femaleness of *maya*, however, is no ordinary quality. It blends in various theories with an under- or overlying maleness. Whereas, however, the female-male communion of Yin-Yang in Chinese Taoism has the feminine as passive and the masculine as active, the Hindu male/female duality reverses the roles: Hindu ascetics turned away from women and the world precisely because they were so active, and that kind of activity—that *karma*—was what bound you to the wheel for ever. In the major theories of the cosmos, the male principle called Shiva or Purusha is perceived as inert and uninvolved, while the female principle of Shakti or Prakriti is marvellously involved, the Cosmic Witch or the triple-goddess of Fate, spinning, spinning, spinning the world and the lives of all beings in that world.

The Cosmic Female has something of the qualities of a spider, spinning from her own essence the three twining strands from which all things are constituted. In the *Bhagavad-Gita*, Krishna has quite a lot to say about these strands, beginning: 'There are three states in nature, three strands, three *gunas*—and they come from me. They are the virtuous *sattva*, the passionate *rajas*, and the dark and heavy *tamas*. They are in me, but I am not in them. They serve to snare and delude the whole world, which cannot perceive that I lie beyond them, unchanging and undying. Out of these *gunas* is woven my *maya*, a power that is hard to escape. Only those that trust me can get beyond that uncanny force.'

So, in essence, there is an over-being—usually conceived as male—who contains or emanates an active female force, or this over-being contains both a male passive element and a female active element. The picture varies from sect to sect, but whatever the permutations, the power of *maya* spun out of the divine background of the universe is feminine and fertile, bursting with the forms of life and time. Of it, Heinrich Zimmer observes:

Maya is existence: both the world of which we are aware, and ourselves who are contained in the growing and dissolving environment, growing and dissolving in our turn. At the same time, Maya is the supreme power that generates and animates the display: the dynamic aspect of the universal substance. Thus it is at once, effect (the cosmic flux), and cause (the creative power). In the latter regard it is known as Shakti, 'Cosmic Energy.' The noun *śakti* is from the root *śak*, signifying 'to be able, to be possible.' *Śakti* is power, ability, capacity, faculty, strength, energy, prowess, regal power; the power of composition, poetic power, genius; the power or signification of a word or term . . . *śakti* is the female organ; *śakti* is the active power of a deity and is regarded, mythologically, as his goddess-consort and queen. Maya-Shakti is personified as the world-protecting, feminine, maternal side of the Ultimate Being, and as such, stands for the spontaneous, loving acceptance of life's tangible reality . . . She is the creative joy of life.[68]

Particularly in the Tantric view of things, where men enamoured of ascetic power were either less common or less inclined to turn their backs completely on her blandishments. In Tantra, the goal has not necessarily been, as in other disciplines, to escape the snare of *maya*, but to understand it—to grasp how it is woven. Tantra means 'loom'.

The concept of the *gunas* derives from *Sankhya* philosophy, one of the earliest systems anywhere in the world to offer a comprehensive 'map' of reality. The first principle in Sankhya is *Purusha*, according to Theos Bernard 'the soul of the universe . . . which breathes life into matter'. The word means 'Person', and is male, while the second principle is *Prakriti* or, in effect, 'Mother Nature', the seat of all manifestation. *Prakriti* consists of three constituents, as follows:

Sattva-guna ('the real thread'): responsible for the lightness in all things, for the upward movement of fire and the blowing of the wind. It is an unruffled kind of force and leads to balance or equilibrium in nature. It can manifest as light, and could be called the spiritual aspect of the material world—the nearest that matter can get to the sublime.

Rajas-guna ('the coloured or passionate thread'): responsible for action and excitement, for change and development. It gives the force to wind and fire, and could be called vitality.

Tamas-guna ('the dark thread'): responsible for obstruction and binding, for pulling down where *sattva* raises up and *rajas* whirls around. It resists motion, is heavy and inert. It manifests as darkness, and could be called ignorance.

The yogic interpretation of these three Sankhya concepts is aptly outlined by Alain Daniélou as follows:

The centrifugal force, known as darkness or inertia (*tamas*), is the power that aims at preventing concentration. It is obscurity, since dispersion of energy leads to darkness just as concentration of energy is light . . . The balance of *sattva* and *tamas*, of the centripetal and the centrifugal, of cohesion and dispersion, of light and darkness, gives birth to the third tendency, the revolving tendency, known as 'activity' or 'multiplicity' (*rajas*). It is the source of the endless variety of the forms of the manifest universe. From *rajas*, from the revolving tendency, comes all motion, all rhythmic division of the continua of space and time, all cerebration or mental activity that is rhythmic division of the thought continuum. This third tendency is the process through which creation in its endless variety of forms takes place in the divine mind . . . Though fundamentally distinct, the three qualities are inseparable and cannot exist without each other . . . The word *guna* itself seems to have meant originally 'part of the whole' or, more concretely, one of the filaments constituting a rope.[69]

Only one additional aspect of *maya* remains to be accounted for: that the divine, whatever name or form is given to it, whatever the theory used to describe it, gets a kind of enjoyment or satisfaction from this creative kaleidoscopic magic. Sometimes that enjoyment is symbolized as Vishnu dreaming as he lies on the cosmic snake, but more often it is called *lila* or *lilamaya*—the play of the gods. Conceived in this way, there is every reason for Vishnu to smile as he gets ready to explain his *maya* to Narada—because for Vishnu it is fun.

Lila is play, sport, pastime, diversion, amusement, the playful games of a lover, child's play (in both the literal and the figurative senses), mere appearance, dissimulation, disguise, charm, grace . . . Gods like Krishna have all of these, as they play their flutes, toy with the women who herd the cattle, or persuade an Aryan prince into battle. Divine sport, however, is a serious matter for mortals caught up in it, and the essence of yoga (whatever form it takes) is to see God's joke from God's point of view.

15. PRANA and PRANAYAMA

> Homage to *prana*, breath of life,
> Because the whole cosmos obeys it.
> It has become lord of all,
> And all things are based on it.
>
> Homage to you, breath of life,
> To your thunder, your lightning and your rain . . .
> When *prana* bespatters this mighty earth with rain,
> The cattle bellow the greatness of their share.
>
> Homage to you, breath of life,
> Both when you come and when you go . . .
> Home to you, breath of life,
> When breathing in and breathing out . . . .
>
> *Prana*, don't turn your back on me.
> You will be none other than me.
> Like an embryo in the waters
> I will bind you inside me,
> That I may live!

These verses are from the *Atharva-veda*, which dates back at least three thousand years.[70] It is the fourth and most magically inclined of the Vedas and also the one that is most in tune with the non-Aryan sources from which so much of yoga has developed. The verses quoted are only four among twenty-six that the magicians' *Veda* offers up to what Hiriyanna in 1932 characterized rather graphically as 'deified breath'.[71]

Prana is thus one of the most demonstrably ancient of the key concepts of yoga, and is also one whose essential character has remained the least changed—or perhaps it might be better to say the least evolved. We can for example compare the Vedic verses with the following from B.K.S. Iyengar's *Light on Pranayama*, probably the most detailed book on the subject ever published in English, which came out in 1981:

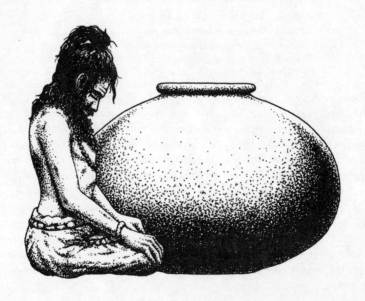

It is as difficult to explain Prāṇa as it is to explain God. Prāṇa is the energy permeating the universe at all levels. It is physical, mental, intellectual, sexual, spiritual and cosmic energy. All vibrating energies are prāṇa. All physical energies such as heat, light, gravity, magnetism and electricity are also prāṇa. It is the hidden or potential energy in all beings, released to the fullest extent in time of danger. It is the prime mover of all activity. It is energy which creates, protects and destroys. Vigour, power, vitality, life and spirit are all forms of prāṇa.[72]

Iyengar points out that in the *Upanishads*, *prana* is equated with *atman*, the innermost non-physical self, while Georg Feuerstein observes that it has been seen as the pervasive stuff out of which the *sukshma-sharira* or subtle physical body is formed. It is something of a rogue term in the systems of yoga, or as Feuerstein puts it: 'Although speculations about this life force reach far back into the vedic [*sic*] age, none of the classical Sanskrit works seem to contain an even approximately precise and satisfactory definition of this important concept.'[73] He notes, however, that the *Yoga Vasishtha* calls it *spanda-shakti*, which he translates as 'vibratory force'. This certainly suggests that the life force of yoga is comparable to both the occultists' idea of all things in the universe as vibrations and the physicists' theories of the cosmos as a kind of rhythmic dance of matter and energy. If it were as 'simple' as that, however, *prana* would be everything, whereas it is clearly *not* everything but a power that operates on everything and is particularly linked with living things. At the same time, however, Swami Vivekananda can say of *prana*:

This opens to us the door to almost unlimited power. Suppose, for instance, a man understood the Prana perfectly, and could control it, what power on earth would not be his? He would be able to move the sun and stars out of their places, to control everything in the universe, from the atoms to the biggest suns, because he would control the Prana. This is the end and aim of Pranayama. When the Yogi becomes perfect, there will be nothing in nature not under his control. If he orders the gods or the souls of the departed to come, they will come at his bidding. All the forces of nature will obey him as slaves. When the ignorant see these powers of the Yogi, they call them the miracles.[74]

It need come as no surprise, therefore, that the first overt enthusiasts for yoga were not the priestly brahmins with their hymns and rituals but the kshatriyas, warriors and governors who appreciated raw power when they met it. *Raja-yoga* is 'the yoga of kings', 'the royal yoga' or 'the king of yoga', and in its very name enshrines the position of the kshatriya princes who developed it. Krishna, himself such a prince, states in the *Gita* that he first explained the yogic truths to Vivasvat the

Sun, who passed them to Manu the first man, who in turn passed them on to King Ikshvaku: 'So the tradition was handed down, and the royal rishis learned it.' Further on he adds, 'I am the sun that shines on the other side of darkness. One who closes all the gates of the body and, keeping a steady mind, centres the energy of life—the *prana*—between his brows, goes to the supreme one.'[75]

In both physical and mystical terms, therefore, nothing is of greater interest to the traditional yogi than *prana*, the breath of life that is more than the breath of life. It is also small wonder that, when yoga teachers talk to their students about the control of this force (which in the West they sometimes call 'bio-energy' rather than simply 'life force') they insist that its most obvious incarnation is in breathing; but to think of *prana* as no more than breath is to be hopelessly mistaken about its significance in the scheme of things. It is seen as the mover and shaker of all things.

Among the classical *darshanas* or philosophies of ancient India, the Yoga of Patanjali and the Sankhya of Kapila are conventionally yoked together as two aspects of the same thing: the nature of the world and what to do about understanding and coming to terms with it. Sankhya provides the general understanding, while Yoga provides the techniques for coming to terms with life and death. In this context, we can talk about a Yoga with a capital Y, because it is the name of an explicitly identified system, whereas in wider contexts it is probably wiser to think of yoga and the various yogas with a small 'y', just as science normally has a small 's'.

Prana appears in Patanjali in relation to *pranayama*, which is the fourth of his eight limbs. Controlling the *prana* for him is a matter of rhythm and regulation: breathing in, holding the breath in, breathing out, holding the breath out, relating the breath to different parts of the body, choosing how long the periods of breathing and retention should be, and regulating the lengths of time by number. In later treatises, particularly those linked with Tantra and hatha-yoga, this rudimentary description is enlarged into a complex interrelationship of life-force, breathing, channels called *nadis* along which pranic currents pass, and the raising of the kundalini, etc. Patanjali, however, says nothing about such things, and appears to be primarily concerned with *pranayama* as one of a cluster of devices for stilling first the body then the mind.

Rather surprisingly, *prana* does not appear at all in the list of 25 primary constituents of the cosmos in Kapila's *Sankhya*, the philosophical partner of Patanjali's Yoga, a system that Theos Bernard has characterized as 'the oldest school of Hindu Philosophy, for it is the first attempt to harmonize the philosophy of the Vedas through reason'.[76] The male and female principles, the elements and many other important features of Hindu thought are there, but not the mysterious life-force.

The basic phases of Hindu breath-control do, however, offer us a clue as to what may be going on. *Puraka* or inhalation and *rechaka* or exhalation are straightforward, but the third term, *kumbhaka*, contains an interesting metaphor. The word means 'potting'—that is, retaining or capping breath as if it were in a sealed pot, jar or bottle. This at first sight seems to be a vivid metaphor for what happens when air enters the lungs and bronchi, etc., but is much more than that, because the physical equipment was not the primary concern of the yogis. They have argued that *prana* actually exists in five forms: *prana* proper, which is associated with inhalation and the chest area; *apana*, which is associated with exhalation and the abdominal area, and with the output of semen, urine, and faeces; *vyana*, which circulates the life force through the entire body; *samana*, which is linked with digestion; and *udana*, which is associated with speech. This is an entirely different geography of bodily airs from Western anatomy and physiology, and has to be accepted and interpreted as such. It suggests, before all else, that the prana that is 'potted' enters the pot of the whole person and not just the containers we call the lungs.

This, I suspect, can be tied to an ancient metaphor that was made particularly well known by the south Indian thinker Gaudapada, one of the major exponents of the Vedanta philosophy, in the seventh century. Basing his theories on the *Upanishads* and later Buddhism, Gaudapada taught *advaita*, the concept that the universe (and each one of us) is 'non-dual', and to illustrate this he compared each of us to jars, pots or bottles. A jar has solidity, separating the air inside from the air outside and making them seem like distinct objects. The two airs, however, are not distinct, as can be seen when the jar breaks, and the two are united again, to be obviously the one condition that they always were in the first place. The analogical air for Gaudapada is the *atman*, and the term 'atman' is itself a word for air or breath (as also in the Greek 'atmosphere').

What we appear to be dealing with here is Hiriyanna's 'deified breath', the idea of a primordial breath-soul that powerfully dominated early Hindu thinking and split into two components: the picture of the air beyond air (*atman*), the ultimate spirit of the universe, and the concept of *prana* as a vital physical force. In both, there is a perception of 'potting' or containerizing—philosophically, the enclosing of spirit in matter; physiologically, the in-flow and out-flow of the life force through mouth and nose. The first is an image of the natural state of things, while the second is a dynamic activity through which everyday life and one's mental balance can be improved if one learns to process the *prana* properly, and to 'pot' it—or 'bind' it, as the *Atharva-veda* puts it—for greater lengths of time.

The splitting of the primordial image of something in a pot or jar serves to conceal the existence of a basic ancient idea that a single air-like substance permeates everything. This is not unlike other more or less magical conceptions in various parts of the world of a vital energy or force connected with important people, places and activities. For the Melanesians it is *mana*, among the Sioux it is *wakan*, the Iroquois call it *orenda*, the Romans had a concept of *numen*, the Greeks of *charisma*, and so forth. In Latin and Western terms, the word 'spirit' is probably the most sophisticated but by no means the most clear-cut of such conceptions. It is inherent in all such terms that, like *prana*, they are even harder to pin down and define than words like 'religion', 'yoga', 'philosophy', and the like. This appears to be because they are so ancient and basic, so all-enveloping and therefore diffuse. It is curious that nineteenth-century science, in order to have a substance that underlies everything else in the universe, took an ancient Greek term *aither* and turned it into 'ether'. The ether is now a discredited scientific concept, but among occultists it is still viable, especially in expressions like 'the etheric body'—not far removed in principle from the subtle body of the Hindus, which is conceived as formed out of *prana*.

I am not arguing here that *prana* 'is the same as' all these other concepts, only that they have something in common. Since they belong to systems of thought and cosmology that are far removed from each other in time and place, they can hardly be brought neatly into alignment with each other. But they can hardly be left totally distinct from each other either. In all such conceptual systems, the basic charge appears to relate to heightened life, and certainly the purpose of *pranayama* is to heighten the quality of life along yogic lines. By controlled breathing, the yogi sought to develop the capacity of his body to hold more *prana*, and so feed the spirit better, making the inner microcosm and the outer macrocosm one by a proper use of the life force itself.

If this is a reasonably satisfactory 'anthropological' explanation of *prana* (*pra ana*, 'the nourishing breath'), in what sense can it be said to exist? Broadly, like *mana* and *charisma*, etc., we can follow Carl Gustav Jung and say that they are 'psychologically real' to the people who use them. This is saying quite a lot, because something that has psychological reality can serve as a turbine to generate all sorts of things, or as a focus to permit all sorts of thoughts. It is not, however, a satisfying answer either for the yogi or the scientist, because the yogi is sure, within his frame of reference, that *prana* is objectively real, and the scientist within his or her frame of reference needs to decide on whether there is in the physical universe a physical element or process that corresponds to the concept, just as a physical current corresponds to the concept 'electricity'.

My own suspicion is that there is no physical entity as such that we can call *prana*, in any sense that Western science could accept and experiment with, and I am drawn to this conclusion not just by the preceding arguments but by the way Iyengar himself describes *pranayama* in his book:

Prāṇāyāma is not just automatic habitual breathing to keep body and soul together. Through the abundant intake of oxygen by its disciplined techniques, subtle chemical changes take place in the sādhaka's body. The practice of āsanas removes the obstructions which impede the flow of prāṇa, and the practice of prāṇāyāma regulates the flow of prāṇa throughout the body. It also regulates all the sādhaka's thoughts, desires and actions, gives poise and the tremendous will-power needed to become a master of oneself.[77]

Here East meets West head on, and the result is an inevitable hybrid language of explanation. 'Oxygen' and 'chemical changes' rub shoulders with *prana*, *asana*, and *sadhak*; the language of science and medicine co-occurs with the language of yoga in a way which very nearly re-defines *prana* as 'oxygen'.

It is necessary but not at all easy to yoke the terminology of yoga and science together, and make them work as a team. Where, for example, *prana* is a millennially ancient and diffuse term that succeeds because it is so comprehensive, 'oxygen' is hardly two hundred years old, and is a tightly delineated term for one of many gases of which the ancient world, East and West, was entirely unaware. Because, however, Western science is such a powerful explanatory system; because it is experimentally built up and can demonstrate its assumptions and techniques in the everyday world with such devastating effect; because tankers laden with liquid oxygen thunder most physically past our doors, any book that ties yogic and scientific terms together runs the risk of finally conceding the ground to science as a means of 'explaining' yoga.

Which is probably necessary; I am doing just that a lot of the time in this book, using the terms and techniques of linguistic science and of anthropology and sociology. We have to be careful, though, not to throw the yogic baby out with this particular bathwater, as for example when we simply glide over ancient Hindu explanations and descriptions in favour of more comfortable and workable Western scientific explanations and descriptions. It is so much easier, in the end, to discuss breath control in terms of oxygen and the cardio-vascular system than to talk about *pranayama* in terms of *prana, asana,* and *sadhaks.* But if we are to be true to yoga, we have to be true to its frame of reference, in which case the effort has to be made, as Iyengar seeks to make it, to let yoga be itself while science is also itself.

What we need for this, and do not yet have, is a theory which does more than cobble East and West together. Instead, whether one calls such a theory yogic or scientific or both, it should unite these two distinct systems by transcending them both, by seeing them as part of a greater whole. To do that, our theory must be a theory of human culture that treats yoga and science with equal respect as products of different civilizations that are trying in distinct and complementary ways to solve the basic puzzles of existence. In the process, it could also harmonize science and the occult, as distinct frames of references or *darshanas* that work in different ways for different people, or for the same person at different times.

The two books of B.K.S. Iyengar are moves in this direction, developed in great detail by a Hindu determined to express his art and convictions in ways which the West can understand and that make sense in a world where hospitals, colleges, and other institutions are constructed on a basis of Western science and technology. Iyengar follows Ernest Wood in insisting that the West take yoga seriously, as a vast and valuable human enterprise. I only ask that we move one step further, and take yoga seriously on its own terms, with its own terms, and not risk failing to understand it by seeing it *only* through the lens of either Western science or Western occultism or indeed Western health-and-fitness programmes.

Prana and *pranayama* make excellent cases in point, because there is so much evidence of their potency. As Dasgupta put it so vividly as long ago as 1927, dealing with breath control at its most impressive: 'With the suspension of the respiratory process the body remains in a state of suspended animation, without any external signs of life. The heart ceases to beat, there is neither taking in of food nor evacuation of any sort, there is no movement of the body . . . I have myself seen a case where the yogin stayed in this condition for nine days.'[78]

That is the ultimate in pranayamic challenges, perhaps, certainly as far as the world of physiology is concerned, but it is not the core of the matter as far as yoga is concerned. That core assumption, however expressed, is that there is a fluidity in the universe, a quality that runs everywhere, sponsoring and sustaining life and incarnated in many forms that have specific names like 'oxygen' and 'electricity'. It is a principle more than a pragmatic fact, but without that principle all the candles of the cosmos, all the stars and all the little lives of humankind would have gone out, one by one, long ago.

That is *prana*, and it is pure magic.

NOTES AND REFERENCES

1 Robert E. Hume, *The Thirteen Principal Upanishads* (Oxford University Press, 1921; 1975 reprint), p. 73.
2 Juan Mascaró, *The Bhagavad Gita* (Penguin, 1962), p. 70.
3 Swami Vivekananda, *Raja Yoga* (Advaita Ashrama, Calcutta, 1962 impression), pp. 222, 231–2.
4 Alain Daniélou, *Yoga: The Method of Re-Integration* (Johnson: London, 1949), p. 36.
5 Daniélou, above, p. 38.
6 Georg Feuerstein, *Textbook of Yoga* (Rider, 1975), p. 102.
7 Benjamin Walker, 'Yoga', *Encyclopaedia of the Unexplained*, ed. Richard Cavendish, consultant J.B. Rhine (Routledge & Kegan Paul, 1974), pp. 280–1.
8 B.K.S. Iyengar, *Light on Yoga* (George Allen & Unwin, 1966), p. 62.
9 Daniélou, above (4), p. 161.
10 Daniélou, above (4), p. 37.
11 Iyengar, above (8), p. 40.
12 Georg Feuerstein, *The Essence of Yoga* (Rider, 1974), p. 92.
13 Louis Fischer, *Gandhi: His Life and Message for the World* (New American Library, 1954), p. 55.
14 *The Longman Dictionary of the English Language* (1984).
15. A.L. Basham, *The Wonder that was India* (Sidgwick & Jackson, 1967), p. 160.
16 Swami Vivekananda, *Jnana Yoga* (Advaita Ashrama, Calcutta, 1964 impression), p. viii.
17 Swami Vivekananda, *Karma Yoga* (Advaita Ashrama, Calcutta, 1963 impression), p. 23.
18 Iyengar, above (8), p. 34.
19 Vivekananda, above (3), pp. 72–3.
20 Ernest Wood, *Yoga* (Penguin, 1959), p. 176.
21 Geoffrey Parrinder, *Sex in the World's Religions* (Sheldon Press, 1980), p. 52.
22 Alain Daniélou, *Hindu Polytheism* (Pantheon Books [Random House], 1964), p. 6.
23 Basham, above (15), p. 335.

24 Geoffrey Parrinder, *Avatar and Incarnation* (Oxford University Press, 1982), p. 17.

25 Sampurnanand, *Evolution of the Hindu Pantheon* (Bharatiya Vidya Bhavan [Bombay], 1963), p. 67.

26 Agehananda Bharati, 'Hindu Scholars, Germany and the Third Reich', *Quest* magazine, India (?1966).

27 Anakchandra Bhayawala, 'Avatars and Darwin', *Bharat Jyoti* (Bombay), Sunday 5 June 1966.

28 Peter Brent, *Godmen of India* (Penguin, 1972), p. 202.

29 Brent, above, p. 207.

30 K.M. Sen, *Hinduism* (Penguin, 1961), p. 91.

31 Basham, above (15), p. 332.

32 Brent, above (28), pp. 169, 171, and 174.

33 Joseph Campbell, *The Masks of God: Oriental Mythology* (Penguin, 1976), pp. 249–50 (first published, Viking Press, 1962).

34 Julian Jaynes, *The Origin of Consciousness in the Breakdown of the Bicameral Mind* (Houghton Mifflin [Boston], 1976).

35 Charles Hampden-Turner, *Maps of the Mind: Charts and Concepts of the Mind and its Labyrinths* (Mitchell Beazley [London] and Macmillan [New York], 1981), esp. Map 21, 'Lying Down with a Horse and a Crocodile: The Papez-MacLean Theory of Brain Evolution', pp. 80–3, discussing the work of James W. Papez and Paul D. MacLean.

36 Shree Purohit Swami, *Bhagwan Shree Patanjali, Aphorisms of Yoga* (Faber & Faber, 1938).

37 Gopi Krishna, *Kundalini* (London, 1971), p. 66.

38 Swami Gnaneswarananda, 'Lessons in Meditation', in *Meditation* (Rama Krishna Vedanta Centre [London], 1972), p. 73.

39 Feuerstein, above (12), p. 190.

40 Basham, above (15), p. 329.

41 Peter Rendel, *Introduction to the Chakras* (Aquarian Press, 1974; revised 1979), pp. 9–10 and 77.

42 Feuerstein, above (6), pp. 165–7.

43 Rendel, above (41), p. 13.

44 Swami Satchidananda, 'Awakening the Kundalini', *Journal of the Scottish Yoga Association* 14 (January 1979).

45 Feuerstein, above (6), p. 168.

46 M. Hiriyanna, *Outline of Indian Philosophy* (George Allen & Unwin, 1932), p. 163.

47 Hiriyanna, above, pp. 182–3.

48 Alain Daniélou, above (22), p. 6.

49 Gita Mehta, *Karma Cola: Marketing the Mystic East* (Collins/Fontana, 1981), pp. 30 & 34.

50 Vivekananda, above (3), p. 80.

51 Vivekananda, above (3), p. 81.

52 Swami Ashokananda, 'Before You Sit in Meditation', in above (38), p. 2.

53 Eugene Herrigel, *The Method of Zen* (Vintage Books, 1974 [Random House

original, 1960]), pp. 19–20.

54 Jane Thomson, 'Outline of a Guru', in *JSYA*, above (44), 10 (January 1978).

55 Brent, above (28), p. 16.

56 B.K.S. Iyengar, 'How Yoga Transformed Me', in *JSYA* above (44), 10 (January 1978).

57 Brent, above (28), p. 55.

58 Vivekananda, above (17), pp. 1–4.

59 Heinrich Zimmer, *The Art of Indian Asia: Its Mythology and Transformations*, completed and edited by Joseph Campbell (Pantheon Books [Random House], 1955; 2nd edition 1960), pp. 129–30.

60 Basham, above (15), pp. 324–5.

61 Wood, above (20), p. 210.

62 Wood, above (20), p. 9.

63 Wood, above (20), p. 210.

64 Wood, above (20), pp. 210–11.

65 Feuerstein, above (6), p. 152.

66 Wood, above (20), p. 192.

67 Feuerstein, above (6), pp. 153–4. Cf. also Feuerstein above (12), pp. 180–1. Cf. also Zimmer, below, p. 141.

68 Heinrich Zimmer, *Myths and Symbols in Indian Art and Civilization*, ed. Joseph Campbell (Pantheon Books [Random House], 1946), p. 25.

69 Daniélou, above (22), pp. 22–4.

70 *Atharva-veda* XI. iv. My version.

71 Hiriyanna, above (46), p. 41.

72 B.K.S. Iyengar, *Light on Pranayama* (George Allen & Unwin, 1981), p. 12.

73 Feuerstein, above (12), p. 96.

74 Vivekananda, above (3), p. 38.

75 Tom McArthur, *Yoga and the Bhagavad-Gita* (Aquarian Press, 1986), pp. 91 and 95–6.

76 Theos Bernard, *Hindu Philosophy* (Philosophical Library [New York], 1947), p. 66.

77 Iyengar, above (72), p. 14.

78 S.N. Dasgupta, *Hindu Mysticism* (Chicago, 1927), p. 75.

Index